T0259618

INTERVENTIONAL CARDIOLOGY CLINICS

www.interventional.theclinics.com

Editor-in-Chief

MATTHEW J. PRICE

Transradial Angiography and Intervention

April 2015 • Volume 4 • Number 2

Editor

SUNIL V. RAO

ELSEVIER

1600 John F. Kennedy Boulevard • Suite 1800 • Philadelphia, Pennsylvania, 19103-2899

http://www.theclinics.com

INTERVENTIONAL CARDIOLOGY CLINICS Volume 4, Number 2
April 2015 ISSN 2211-7458, ISBN-13: 978-0-323-35977-1

Editor: Adrianne Brigido
Developmental Editor: Barbara Cohen-Kligerman

Interventional Cardiology Clinics (ISSN 2211-7458) is published quarterly by Elsevier Inc., 360 Park Avenue South, New York, NY 10010-1710. Months of issue are January, April, July, and October. Subscription prices are USD 195 per year for US individuals, USD 305 for US institutions, USD 130 per year for US students, USD 230 per year for Canadian individuals, USD 375 for Canadian institutions, USD 150 per year for Canadian students, USD 295 per year for international individuals, USD 375 for international institutions, and USD 150 per year for international students. To receive student/resident rate, orders must be accompanied by name of affiliated institution, date of term, and the *signature* of program/ residency coordinator on institution letterhead. Orders will be billed at individual rate until proof of status is received. Foreign air speed delivery is included in all *Clinics* subscription prices. All prices are subject to change without notice. **POSTMASTER:** Send address changes to *Interventional Cardiology Clinics*, Elsevier Health Sciences Division, Subscription Customer Service, 3251 Riverport Lane, Maryland Heights, MO 63043. **Customer Service: Telephone: 1-800-654-2452** (U.S. and Canada); **1-314-447-8871** (outside U.S. and Canada). **Fax: 1-314-447-8029. E-mail: journalscustomerservice-usa@elsevier. com** (for print support); **journalsonlinesupport-usa@elsevier.com** (for online support).

Reprints. For copies of 100 or more of articles in this publication, please contact the Commercial Reprints Department, Elsevier Inc., 360 Park Avenue South, New York, NY 10010-1710. Tel.: 212-633-3874; Fax: 212-633-3820; E-mail: reprints@elsevier.com.

CONTRIBUTORS

EDITOR-IN-CHIEF

MATTHEW J. PRICE, MD
Assistant Professor, Scripps Translational
Science Institute; Director of the Cardiac
Catheterization Laboratory, Scripps Green
Hospital; Division of Cardiovascular Diseases,
Scripps Clinic, La Jolla, California

EDITOR

SUNIL V. RAO, MD, FACC, FSCAI
Associate Professor with Tenure, Duke
University Medical Center; Section Chief,
Cardiology, Durham VA Medical Center,
Durham, North Carolina

AUTHORS

CARLOS E. ALFONSO, MD
Cardiac Catheterization Laboratory,
Cardiovascular Division; Assistant Professor of
Medicine, Department of Medicine, University
of Miami Hospital, University of Miami Miller
School of Medicine, Miami, Florida

VINAY ARORA, MD
Section of Cardiology, University of Illinois
Hospital and Health Sciences System; Section
of Cardiology, Jesse Brown VA Medical
Center, Chicago, Illinois

OLIVIER F. BERTRAND, MD, PhD
Quebec Heart-Lung Institute, Quebec City,
Quebec, Canada

MAURICIO G. COHEN, MD, FACC, FSCAI
Director, Cardiac Catheterization Laboratory,
Cardiovascular Division; Associate Professor
of Medicine, Department of Medicine,
University of Miami Hospital, University of
Miami Miller School of Medicine, Miami,
Florida

JOHN COPPOLA, MD, FACC, FSCAI
Department of Cardiology, NYU Langone
Medical Center, New York, New York

OLIVIER COSTEROUSSE, PhD
Quebec Heart-Lung Institute, Quebec City,
Quebec, Canada

IAN C. GILCHRIST, MD, FSCAI
Professor of Medicine, Division of Cardiology
Heart and Vascular Institute, Pennsylvania
State University College of Medicine, Hershey,
Pennsylvania

RAJIV GULATI, MD, PhD
Associate Professor of Medicine, Division of
Cardiovascular Diseases, Mayo Clinic,
Rochester, Minnesota

SASKO KEDEV, MD, PhD, FESC, FACC
Medical Faculty, Professor of Medicine
(Cardiology); Director, University Clinic of
Cardiology, University of St. Cyril and
Methodius, Skopje, Macedonia

SAMIR B. PANCHOLY, MD, FACC, FSCAI
Associate Professor and Program Director,
Department of Cardiology, The Wright Center
for Graduate Medical Education, The
Commonwealth Medical College, Scranton,
Pennsylvania

MEET PATEL, MD
Section of Cardiology, University of Illinois
Hospital and Health Sciences System; Section
of Cardiology, Jesse Brown VA Medical
Center, Chicago, Illinois

TEJAS M. PATEL, MD, FACC, FSCAI, FESC
Chairman, Apex Heart Institute; Professor and
Head, Department of Cardiology, Sheth V.S.
General Hospital, Smt. N.H.L. Municipal
Medical College, Ahmedabad, India

ALBERTO BARRIA PEREZ, MD
Quebec Heart-Lung Institute, Quebec City, Quebec, Canada

GUILLAUME PLOURDE, MS
Quebec Heart-Lung Institute, Quebec City, Quebec, Canada

YANN POIRIER, MS
Quebec Heart-Lung Institute, Quebec City, Quebec, Canada

GORAN RIMAC, MS
Quebec Heart-Lung Institute, Quebec City, Quebec, Canada

KINTUR SANGHVI, MD, FACC, FSCAI
Director of Transradial Program, Department of Interventional Cardiology and Endovascular Medicine, Deborah Heart and Lung Center, Browns Mills, New Jersey; Associate Professor of Medicine, Philadelphia College of Osteopathic Medicine, Philadelphia, Pennsylvania

SAURABH SANON, MD
Fellow, Division of Cardiovascular Diseases, Mayo Clinic, Rochester, Minnesota

SANJAY SHAH, MD
Director of Cardiology, Apex Heart Institute; Associate Professor, Department of Cardiology, Sheth V.S. General Hospital, Smt. N.H.L. Municipal Medical College, Ahmedabad, India

ADHIR R. SHROFF, MD, MPH
Section of Cardiology, University of Illinois Hospital and Health Sciences System; Section of Cardiology, Jesse Brown VA Medical Center, Chicago, Illinois

CONTENTS

Radial Artery Access, Hemostasis, and Radial Artery Occlusion   121
Samir B. Pancholy, Sanjay Shah, and Tejas M. Patel

> Radial artery access is usually achieved using a micropuncture system. Hydro-philic introducers are used to improve comfort, probably by reducing spasm. A vasodilator cocktail should be administered to prevent severe spasm and anticoagulation; usually, unfractionated heparin is administered to prevent sub-sequent radial artery occlusion (RAO). Hemostasis at the radial artery puncture site is easily achievable by local compression. Application of local compression frequently leads to interruption of radial artery flow and subsequent occlusion. Careful attention to maintenance of radial artery patency during hemostatic compression has been shown to decrease the risk of RAO without increasing access-related bleeding complications.

Strategies to Traverse the Arm and Chest Vasculature   127
Tejas M. Patel, Sanjay Shah, and Samir B. Pancholy

> This article discusses different methods of working through arm and chest vasculature to increase the success rate of the transradial approach (TRA). Despite lower rates of bleeding and vascular complications as compared with the transfemoral approach, adoption of the TRA has been slow, particu-larly because of higher failure rates. Anatomic complexities of arm and chest vasculature play an important role in cases of TRA failure. Using a simple frame-work to classify the anatomic or functional problem and approaching these challenges in a logical sequence should facilitate management and increase the success rate for TRA.

Diagnostic and Guide Catheter Selection and Manipulation for Radial Approach   145
Carlos E. Alfonso and Mauricio G. Cohen

> Transradial catheterization and percutaneous coronary interventions have mul-tiple advantages, including reduced bleeding risk, reduced length of stay and costs, and increased patient comfort. Transradial catheterization and interven-tions requires the acquisition of various additional skill sets including radial arterial puncture, the ability to navigate the upper extremity vasculature, and understanding catheter selection and coronary engagement technique. Although standard femoral catheter shapes perform adequately from the left or right radial approach for coronary angiography, for percutaneous coro-nary intervention guide catheter support is critical. This article summarizes some practical learning points pertaining to navigating the upper extremity vasculature, and understanding catheter selection and coronary engagement technique.

Most radial arteries cannot accommodate 7- and 8-French Introducer sheaths for large-bore percutaneous coronary intervention without overstretch. In addition to being uncomfortable, radial artery overstretch is associated with spasm and higher rates of procedure-related radial artery occlusion. Methods for the transradial interventionist to overcome the limitation of radial artery–sheath size mismatch include both sheath-based and sheathless approaches. In this article we discuss a variety of techniques that can be used to minimize radial artery stretch for straightforward and complex coronary procedures.

 Videos of right forearm angiogram demonstrating significant radial artery tortuosity and tortuosity negotiated with 0.014-inch guidewire accompany this article

Despite advances in antithrombotic and antiplatelet therapy, bleeding complications remain an important cause of morbidity and mortality in patients with acute ST segment elevation myocardial infarction (STEMI) undergoing primary percutaneous coronary intervention (PPCI). Many bleeding events are related to the access site. Transradial access (TRA) PPCI is associated with significant reduction in bleeding and vascular complications and reduced cardiac mortality compared with the transfemoral approach (TFA). High-risk patients might particularly benefit from TRA. Radial skills providing procedural times and success rates comparable with those of the TFA are strongly recommended before using this technique in the STEMI PPCI setting.

 Videos of transradial peripheral arterial procedures accompany this article

Increased understanding and increased adoption of transradial catheterization across the world have led to further exploring of radial artery access for transradial endovascular interventions in peripheral artery disease (PAD). This article discusses the advantages and limitations of the transradial approach for endovascular medicine by using case examples, illustrations, and videos. The details about how to use a radial approach for PAD intervention, including tips and tricks, are discussed.

The transradial approach for coronary angiography has become an increasingly used alternative to the conventional transfemoral approach. Decreased access site complications and bleeding, reduced hospital stays and health care costs, and increased patient satisfaction contribute to the attractiveness of this approach. However, operators must be familiar with the distinct complications associated with the transradial approach. In this article, we discuss the common and less common complications of transradial catheterization, prevention strategies, and management options.

This article discusses how learning curves correlate with learning in transradial catheterization. Although learning curves exist in the conversion to transradial approaches, current percutaneous coronary intervention (PCI) procedures are so safe that only surrogate end points such as contrast usage and x-ray exposure show learning effects. Using these surrogates, a learning curve of 30 to 50 patients seems typical to transition cardiologists from transfemoral to transradial PCI. This transition occurs with the immediate benefit of reduced vascular complications and bleeding and without loss of overall procedural success. These measures of safety during learning exist despite difference of procedural volumes.

This article reviews antithrombotic strategies for percutaneous coronary interventions according to the access site and the current evidence with the aim of limiting ischemic complications and preventing radial artery occlusion (RAO). Prevention of RAO should be part of the quality control of any radial program. The incidence of RAO postcatheterization and interventions should be determined initially using the echo-duplex and then frequently assessed using the more cost-effective pulse oximetry technique. Any evidence of higher risk of RAO should prompt internal analysis and multidisciplinary mechanisms to be put in place.

TRANSRADIAL ANGIOGRAPHY AND INTERVENTION

ISSUE OF RELATED INTEREST

Cardiology Clinics, August 2014 (Vol. 32, No. 3)
Coronary Artery Disease
David M. Shavelle, *Editor*
Available at: http://www.cardiology.theclinics.com/

THE CLINICS ARE NOW AVAILABLE ONLINE!

Access your subscription at:
www.theclinics.com

PREFACE

Radial Approach: Fundamental Techniques and Evidence

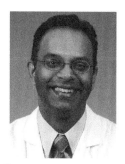

Sunil V. Rao, MD, FACC, FSCAI
Editor

Bleeding is the most common complication of percutaneous coronary intervention (PCI), occurring in up to 10% of patients. A substantial proportion of bleeding is related to the vascular access site, and studies indicate that such complications are associated with increased morbidity, mortality, and costs. These complications are also largely preventable. The most effective strategy to reduce bleeding risk from PCI is to use the radial artery instead of the femoral artery. Transradial PCI is being increasingly adopted, but there is substantial international variation in its use. In particular, certain countries, such as the United States, lag behind other countries, such as India and Japan. This may be due to the lack of concise information on best practices and techniques. There also has been a significant increase in the number of publications on the radial approach examining high-risk subsets and clinical and nonclinical outcomes. Observational and randomized studies have shown that radial access reduces mortality in patients with ST-segment elevation myocardial infarction (STEMI) and reduces hospital length of stay and costs compared with traditional femoral access.

This issue of *Interventional Cardiology Clinics* provides an in-depth examination of relevant transradial topics written by international experts for the practicing interventional cardiologist. The issue includes such topics as radial arterial access, hemostasis and radial artery occlusion; traversing the arm and chest vasculature; and diagnostic and guide catheter selection. Also found in the issue are advanced topics such as sheathless techniques, transradial primary PCI for STEMI, use of radial access for peripheral arterial procedures, and recognition and management of complications. In addition, topics such as the radial learning curve and the interaction between access site and antithrombotic therapy are also explored.

Importantly, each article focuses on practical information that is readily translatable to clinical practice. Taken together, this compendium represents the best contemporary information on radial access, which will contribute to improving the care of patients undergoing PCI.

Sunil V. Rao, MD, FACC, FSCAI
Duke University Medical Center
Durham VA Medical Center
508 Fulton Street (111A)
Durham, NC 27705, USA
E-mail address:
sunil.rao@duke.edu

Intervent Cardiol Clin 4 (2015) ix
http://dx.doi.org/10.1016/j.iccl.2015.01.005
2211-7458/15/$ – see front matter © 2015 Published by Elsevier Inc.

Radial Artery Access, Hemostasis, and Radial Artery Occlusion

Samir B. Pancholy, MD, FACC, FSCAI[a,*], Sanjay Shah, MD[b,c],
Tejas M. Patel, MD, FACC, FSCAI, FESC[b,c]

KEYWORDS

- Access • Hemostasis • Patency • Reaccess

KEY POINTS

- Radial artery access requires dedicated equipment and has a learning curve.
- Counterpuncture technique has a higher first-attempt success rate and seems faster at obtaining radial artery access.
- Using the smallest caliber hydrophilic introducers and administration of vasodilators as well as an adequate dose of unfractionated heparin (UFH) remain best practices.
- Radial artery hemostasis, despite being an apparently simple process and highly efficacious at preventing bleeding complications, has serious implications for radial artery flow and lumen preservation.
- Applying current best practices is the most evidence-based approach to optimal radial hemostasis.

INTRODUCTION

Transradial access (TRA) has been associated with reduction in access site complications[1] and procedure-related cost[2] and is preferred by patients[3] compared with transfemoral access. This review describes the technique and best practices for obtaining radial artery access and the technique of hemostasis and its relationship with postprocedural radial artery occlusion (RAO).

RADIAL ARTERY ACCESS

Patient Selection

Most patients referred for cardiac catheterization or peripheral endovascular procedures are candidates for TRA. In view of extensive microcollateralization and frequent presence of macrocollateral circuits, the forearm arteries do not behave as end arteries and make ideal access sites. Tests for assessment of the presence of macrocollateral circuits have been found to have no utility in triaging patients to or away from TRA.[4] Specific patient subsets deemed less suitable for TRA are limited to patients with scleroderma, due to the risk of diffuse spasm leading to ischemia, and patients with ipsilateral dialysis access.

Patient Set-Up

In a typical catheterization laboratory, the patient is prepped in a supine position, with the right hand gently extended. A variety of drapes covering the arm, exposing the distal forearm, are commercially available and frequently used. An operator may choose to obtain radial artery access with the upper extremity abducted or

S.B. Pancholy is a Consultant for Terumo Corporation (Somerset, NJ). Drs S. Shah and T.M. Patel have nothing to disclose.

[a] Department of Cardiology, The Wright Center for Graduate Medical Education, The Commonwealth Medical College, 501 Madison Avenue, Scranton, PA 18510, USA; [b] Apex Heart Institute, S. G. Road, Ahmedabad 380 054, India; [c] Department of Cardiology, Sheth V.S. General Hospital, Smt. N.H.L. Municipal Medical College, Ellisbridge, Ahmedabad 380 006, India

* Corresponding author. 401 North State Street, Clarks Summit, PA 18411.

E-mail address: pancholys@gmail.com

placed in a supinated position next to the patient's trunk. For left radial access, a similar preparation is sufficient, and arterial puncture is accomplished with the operator standing either on the patient's right side or on the patient's left side. Once the guide wire is placed above the elbow joint, the left upper extremity could be adducted over to the patient's midline and the procedure performed with the operator standing on the patient's right side.

Radial Artery Puncture

After local infiltration with 1 to 2 mL of lidocaine, the radial artery is punctured, ideally 2 to 3 fingerbreadths above the radial styloid process. A micropuncture needle is used in most instances. Either a bare needle or a Teflon-sheathed needle may be used. The traditional anterior puncture technique may be used, where the operator, after puncturing the anterior wall of the radial artery and visualizing bleeding from the needle hub, immobilizes the needle and advances the guide wire (Fig. 1). The other commonly used technique is the counterpuncture technique (Fig. 2), where, after appearance of blood in the needle hub, indicating anterior wall puncture, the needle is advanced through the lumen and the posterior wall is punctured. The needle is then gently withdrawn into the arterial lumen, and the guide wire is advanced once continuous or pulsatile flow of blood is seen. When a Teflon-sheathed needle is used, the inner stylet is removed after needle stabilization and a similar procedure is used. Counterpuncture technique has been shown faster and more likely to succeed at first attempt and has not been associated with an increase in bleeding or RAO.[5]

Arterial Access

After placement of a micropuncture guide wire (0.018-in or 0.021-in) in the radial artery lumen, an introducer sheath is inserted. Hydrophilic-coated introducer sheaths have been associated with less spasm[6] and found easier to remove.[7] After placement of an introducer sheath, a vasodilator cocktail is administered intra-arterially.

Nitrates and/or calcium channel blockers are common ingredients of the vasodilator cocktail; 5000 units of UFH are usually administered to lower the incidence of RAO. UFH can be administered intra-arterially or intravenously with equivalent prophylactic efficacy.[8]

TECHNIQUE OF HEMOSTASIS

Radial artery hemostasis can be achieved fairly easily by local manual compression. The firm and flat base of the radius bone is ideally suitable for compression and in conjunction with a thick-walled structure of the radial artery; bleeding at the puncture site can be stopped by application of modest pressure. Several hemostatic compression practices are prevalent, ranging from manual compression to compression dressings and, recently, the increasing use of circumferential bands capable of applying titratable pressure. All of these modalities are highly effective in achieving hemostasis. The bands allow for patients to be free and ambulate immediately postprocedure.

Caution should be exercised to apply the center point of the bands at the site of arterial puncture (usually proximal to the skin entry site) to prevent bleeding complications when practicing low-pressure hemostasis.

PREVENTION OF RADIAL ARTERY OCCLUSION

RAO is the most frequent structural complication of TRA, with prevalence ranging from 2% to 10%.[9] Several procedural variables affect the occurrence of RAO, including the following:

- Larger-size hardware compared with the radial artery lumen[10]
- Absence of anticoagulation[11]
- Interruption of radial artery flow during and after hemostatic compression[12]

Hemostatic compression using excessive pressure, although increasing the confidence in the hemostatic efficacy, frequently leads to

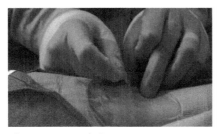

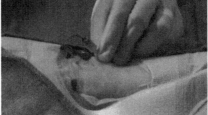

Fig. 1. Anterior puncture technique.

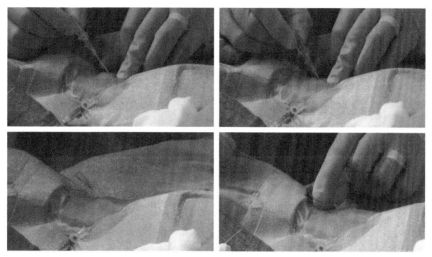

Fig. 2. Counterpuncture technique.

complete cessation of radial artery flow. This, in conjunction with fresh intimal abrasion caused by insertion and removal of hardware, creates an ideal environment for thrombus formation. Transmural thrombus formation is the most common mechanism of RAO.[13] Decreasing the compression pressure to the point of re-establishment of radial artery patency, while maintaining hemostatic efficacy, termed *patent hemostasis*, is associated with an incremental decrease in incidence of RAO.[14,15] This is associated with no increase in bleeding complications. Because radial artery preservation is of paramount importance in view of systemic and progressive nature of atherosclerotic disease and the resultant need for repeat procedures, patent hemostasis has become a core component of

best practices for TRA.[16] The practice of patent hemostasis does not require the use of a specific device and revolves around the fastidious adoption of paying close attention to radial patency at the outset and throughout the duration of hemostatic compression.

The technique of patent hemostasis is as follows (because bands are increasingly used to achieve hemostasis, this protocol describes the technique using a band):

Step 1: After completion of the procedure, apply the hemostatic compression device at the radial access site. Pay careful attention to centering the device to the arterial puncture site (Fig. 3A).

Step 2: Compress the access site by increasing the pressure applied by the band.

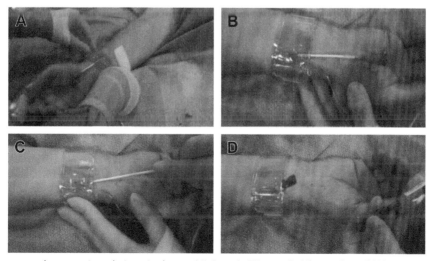

Fig. 3. The patent hemostasis technique is shown. (*A*) Step 1, (*B*) step 2, (*C*) step 3, and (*D*) step 4. See text for details.

Once compression of the subcutaneous tissue is evident, remove the introducer sheath from under the band. Allow the introducer sheath side port to bleed on its way out, to purge the pre-thrombotic contents of the radial artery lumen (see Fig. 3B).

Once the introducer sheath is removed, if the band is providing hemostasis, proceed to step 4. If bleeding is evident at the puncture site, increase the compression pressure given by the band to eliminate all visible bleeding (see Fig. 3C).

Step 4: Gradually decrease the compression pressure in the band until minor bleeding (leakage) is seen at the puncture site, and, once bleeding is seen, increase the pressure just enough to completely eliminate the bleeding (see Fig. 3D).

Step 5: Perform a reverse Barbeau test to assess for presence of antegrade flow in the radial artery. If antegrade flow is present in radial artery (presence of plethysmographic waveform on compression of ipsilateral ulnar artery), leave the band in place. If antegrade flow in radial artery is not present, titrate the pressure to the lowest needed pressure to achieve hemostasis. In the first 10 to 15 minutes of initiating hemostatic compression, due to changes in the dynamic balance of local influences, repeat attempts at achieving the balance of patency and hemostasis frequently succeed, even if the very initial attempt does not.

Step 6: Once optimal hemostatic compression is achieved, continue to monitor the presence of radial artery patency periodically (every 15 minutes) by using reverse Barbeau test. The patient is instructed to report immediately if any bleeding is observed at the site.

If radial artery patency is not achievable at the outset, despite continuous attempts, re-evaluation at 15 minutes and reattempting establishment of patent hemostasis are advised.

RECANALIZATION AFTER RADIAL ARTERY OCCLUSION

RAO in most instances is a result of transmural thrombosis of radial artery lumen due to intimal disruption caused by catheter entry and exit and flow cessation. In 50% to 60% of patients, a freshly occluded radial artery spontaneously recanalizes, with establishment of a stable lumen, at follow-up. Another mechanism suspected of playing a role in immediate postprocedural RAO is severe local spasm. Immediate recanalization after ulnar compression, without distal embolization, observed in a recent study,[17] likely resulted largely from relief of intense local spasm. A recent

randomized evaluation of a precompression vaso-dilator (500 µg nitroglycerin), compared with placebo, showed a significant reduction in 24-hour RAO incidence, further emphasizing the significant role residual spasm might be playing in increasing the probability of RAO.[18]

SUMMARY

Radial artery access requires dedicated equipment and has a learning curve. Counterpuncture technique has a higher first-attempt success rate and seems faster at obtaining radial artery access. Using the smallest caliber hydrophilic introducers and administration of vasodilators as well as an adequate dose of UFH remain best practices. Radial artery hemostasis, despite being an apparently simple process and highly efficacious at preventing bleeding complications, has serious implications for radial artery flow and lumen preservation. Applying current best practices is the most evidence-based approach to optimal radial hemostasis.

REFERENCES

1. Bertrand OF, Bélisle P, Joyal D, et al. Comparison of transradial and femoral approaches for percutaneous coronary interventions: a systematic review and hierarchical Bayesian meta-analysis. Am Heart J 2012;163(4):632–48.
2. Safley DM, Amin AP, House JA, et al. Comparison of costs between transradial and transfemoral percutaneous coronary intervention: a cohort analysis from the Premier research database. Am Heart J 2013;165(3):303–9.
3. Cooper CJ, El-Shiekh RA, Cohen DJ, et al. Effect of transradial access on quality of life and cost of cardiac catheterization: a randomized comparison. Am Heart J 1999;138(3 Pt 1):430–6.
4. Valgimigli M, Campo G, Penzo C, et al, RADAR Investigators. Transradial coronary catheterization and intervention across the whole spectrum of Allen test results. J Am Coll Cardiol 2014;63(18):1833–41.
5. Pancholy SB, Sanghvi KA, Patel TM. Radial artery access technique evaluation trial: randomized comparison of Seldinger versus modified Seldinger technique for arterial access for transradial catheterization. Catheter Cardiovasc Interv 2012;80(2): 288–91.
6. Rathore S, Stables RH, Pauriah M, et al. Impact of length and hydrophilic coating of the introducer sheath on radial artery spasm during transradial coronary intervention: a randomized study. JACC Cardiovasc Interv 2010;3(5):475–83.
7. Saito S, Tanaka S, Hiroe Y, et al. Usefulness of hydrophilic coating on arterial sheath introducer in

transradial coronary intervention. Catheter Cardiovasc Interv 2002;56(3):328–32.

8. Pancholy SB. Comparison of the effect of intra-arterial versus intravenous heparin on radial artery occlusion after transradial catheterization. Am J Cardiol 2009;104(8):1083–5.

9. Kotowycz MA, Dzavík V. Radial artery patency after transradial catheterization. Circ Cardiovasc Interv 2012;5(1):127–33.

10. Saito S, Ikei H, Hosokawa G, et al. Influence of the ratio between radial artery inner diameter and sheath outer diameter on radial artery flow after transradial coronary intervention. Catheter Cardiovasc Interv 1999;46(2):173–8.

11. Spaulding C, Lefèvre T, Funck F, et al. Left radial approach for coronary angiography: results of a prospective study. Cathet Cardiovasc Diagn 1996; 39(4):365–70.

12. Sanmartin M, Gomez M, Rumoroso JR, et al. Interruption of blood flow during compression and radial artery occlusion after transradialcatheterization. Catheter Cardiovasc Interv 2007;70(2):185–9.

13. Pancholy SB. Transradial access in an occluded radial artery: new technique. J Invasive Cardiol 2007;19(12):541–4.

14. Pancholy S, Coppola J, Patel T, et al. Prevention of radial artery occlusion-patent hemostasis evaluation trial (PROPHET study): a randomized comparison of traditional versus patency documented hemostasis after transradial catheterization. Catheter Cardiovasc Interv 2008;72(3):335–40.

15. Cubero JM, Lombardo J, Pedrosa C, et al. Radial compression guided by mean artery pressure versus standard compression with a pneumatic device (RACOMAP). Catheter Cardiovasc Interv 2009; 73(4):467–72.

16. Rao SV, Tremmel JA, Gilchrist IC, et al, Society for Cardiovascular Angiography and Intervention's Transradial Working Group. Best practices for transradial angiography and intervention: a consensus statement from the society for cardiovascular angiography and intervention's transradial working group. Catheter Cardiovasc Interv 2014; 83(2):228–36.

17. Bernat I, Bertrand OF, Rokyta R, et al. Efficacy and safety of transient ulnar artery compression to recanalize acute radial artery occlusion after transradial catheterization. Am J Cardiol 2011;107(11): 1698–701.

18. Dharma S, Kedev S, Patel T, et al. A novel approach to reduce radial artery occlusion after transradial catheterization: postprocedural/prehemostasis intra-arterial nitroglycerin. Catheter Cardiovasc Interv 2014. http://dx.doi.org/10.1002/ccd.25661.

Strategies to Traverse the Arm and Chest Vasculature

Tejas M. Patel, MD, FACC, FSCAI, FESC[a,b,*], Sanjay Shah, MD[a,b], Samir B. Pancholy, MD, FACC, FSCAI[c]

KEYWORDS

- Transradial approach • Percutaneous coronary intervention • Complication • Radial artery spasm
- Perforation • Radial artery loop • Subclavian tortuosity • Subclavian stenosis

---

KEY POINTS

- Despite lower rates of bleeding and vascular complications as compared with the transfemoral approach, adoption of the transradial approach (TRA) has been relatively slow, particularly because of higher failure rates.
- Anatomic complexities of arm and chest vasculature play an important role in cases of TRA failure.
- Understanding these complexities of the vasculature can lead to standardization of solutions for a higher success rate, shorter procedure time, and lower radiation dose.

INTRODUCTION

One challenge of transradial angiography and intervention is that the route to the coronary ostium is potentially far more varied for the radial approach compared with the femoral approach.[1–5] The radial operator is presented with several potential anatomic complexities and variations while traversing through the arm and chest vasculature that typically do not exist for the transfemoral approach. Understanding these complexities of the vasculature can lead to standardization of solutions for a higher success rate, shorter procedure time, and lower radiation dose.[6–12] In this article, an in-depth discussion of radial artery (RA), brachial artery (BA), subclavian artery (SA), and innominate artery (IA) vasculature complexities along with the methods to manage them is described.

Broadly, the arm and chest vascular complexities can be divided into several subsets, including (1) radial artery spasm; (2) variant anatomy, including tortuosity, loops, and anomalous origin of RA; (3) acquired abnormalities including perforations, atherosclerotic lesions, and calcification of RA; (4) tortuosities in the SA and IA region; (5) loops in the SA and IA region; (6) stenosis in the SA and IA region; (7) arteria lusoria; and (8) combined challenges in the SA and IA region (Box 1).[11,12]

An understanding of normal anatomy of this region is necessary to deal with these issues effectively. Moreover, an operator should also have knowledge of and use a variety of techniques to transverse peripheral vessels, using different catheter types and wires. Techniques such as balloon-assisted tracking (BAT) and facility with a spectrum of wires such as those used in angioplasty are important for effective management when these variants are encountered.

Understanding the Anatomy of Arm and Chest Vasculature

The artery that supplies the upper limb continues as a single trunk from its origin down to

---

The authors have nothing to disclose.

[a] Apex Heart Institute, S. G. Road, Ahmedabad 380 054, India; [b] Department of Cardiology, Sheth V.S. General Hospital, Smt. N.H.L. Municipal Medical College, Ellisbridge, Ahmedabad 380 006, India; [c] Department of Cardiology, The Wright Center for Graduate Medical Education, The Commonwealth Medical College, 501 Madison Avenue, Scranton, PA 18510, USA

* Corresponding author. Apex Heart Institute, S. G. Road, Ahmedabad 380 054, India.
E-mail address: tejaspatel@apexheart.in

the elbow. Different regions of the artery have different names, depending on the anatomic landmarks through which they pass. The part of the artery that extends from its aortic origin to the lateral border of the first rib is the SA. Beyond this point, to the lower border of axilla, it is known as the axillary artery. Beyond this point to the bend of the elbow, the artery is known as the BA. The RA commences at the bifurcation of the BA, just below the bend of the elbow, and passes along the radial side of the forearm to the wrist (Fig. 1A). The RA extends from the neck of the radius to the front part of the styloid process. The upper part lies on the medial side of radius and the lower part lies on the bone. The upper part is deep and lies below the muscle (brachioradialis) in most cases. The lower part is superficial, covered by skin and superficial and deep fascia. The RA is slightly smaller in caliber than the ulnar artery. Variations in the course of the RA are common and occur on the order of 14% of patients.[13] Variation in angiogenesis and selective hypertrophy and regression during early fetal development is thought to underlay many of the congenital variations in origin for the RA.[14] In addition, many of the loops seen at angiography represent alternative development in the RA development and are the end result of passage around muscle or tendon bundles by the RA as it eventually enters its common termination point near the base of the wrist. Arterial tortuosity is thought to be more common in the elderly. Like loops, the artery may also appear tortuous if it travels beyond its "normal" course as a congenital variant. Regardless of whether the course of the radial is normal or varies, none of these variations is known to produce disease or ischemia and should be considered a variation of normally functioning anatomy.

Abnormalities in the radial or brachial distribution can occur. One form of iatrogenic disease is brachial stenosis from prior cut down procedures; this should be suspected in any patient who has had a prior ipsilateral brachial cut down in the years before the radial procedure. The radial and brachial can also acquire disease from the typical degenerative disease of atherosclerosis. Although these smaller peripheral arteries are more resistant to atherosclerosis, it is not immune. In its most extreme form, it can be manifested by medial calcific sclerosis also known as Monckeberg arteriosclerosis.[15,16] Unlike arterial spasm that is dynamic, arteriosclerosis and calcium may represent fixed stenosis that may block catheter passage or impede passage from enhanced resistance.

The anatomy differs on the right and left sides for the SA (see Fig. 1B, C). On the right side, the SA arises from the IA. On the left side, it arises from the arch of the aorta. Although the right and left SA differ in length, direction, and their relationship to neighboring structures in their proximal locations, both share common pathways distally as they extend down the forearm. The innominate-aortic arch junction is unique to transradial procedures. Here the catheters and guidewires must take an obtuse angle turn to enter the ascending aorta. In cases of normal anatomy, the turn is smooth and does not pose obstacles to performing diagnostic or interventional procedures. In cases of abnormal anatomy due to dilation, distortion, or arteria lusoria, the procedure requires judicious use of hardware.

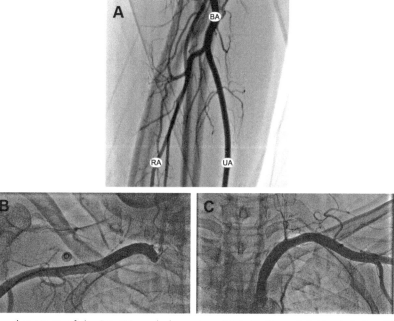

Fig. 1. (*A*) Normal anatomy of the BA, RA, and ulnar artery (UA). (*B*) Normal right subclavian. (*C*) Normal left subclavian.

Tools and Techniques Especially Useful to Overcoming Anatomic Challenges

Operators familiar with interventional techniques have an advantage over diagnostic-only operators because the diagnostic-only operator may not fully appreciate the range of tools available to cross arterial trees. If this is the case, time spent with an interventional colleague to review the local inventory of interventional tools may be worthwhile to maximize the success rate during TRA.

Beyond typical angioplasty techniques, BAT has been described recently to facilitate passage of catheters up vessels that are too narrow for normal passage.[6,17,18] BAT is a technique in which an inflated percutaneous transluminal coronary angioplasty (PTCA) balloon is partially protruded through the distal end of a guide catheter or a diagnostic catheter and deployed at 3 or 6 atm. For 5-F diagnostic or 5-F guide catheters, a balloon diameter of 1.5 mm is recommended. For 6-F guide catheters, a balloon diameter of 2.0 mm is recommended. A balloon length of 15 mm or 20 mm is sufficient. Once the balloon is partially protruded from the distal end of the catheter and deployed, the entire assembly is advanced over a soft-tipped 0.014-in PTCA guidewire, thus allowing smooth and nontraumatic advancement through difficult arm and chest vasculature (Figs. 2 and 3). Anatomic situations that may require BAT include very small caliber RA (diameter <1.5 mm), tortuous RA or BA, severe and resistant RA spasm,

atherosclerotic lesions in RA or BA, complex RA loops, severe subclavian tortuosity, and subclavian stenosis. The key to the BAT technique is its ability to reduce trauma around bends, as noted in Fig. 2, while also nontraumatically encouraging catheter passage up small vessels with a soft leading edge.

Some newer peripheral wires also may provide similar benefits in markets where they are available. Products such as the Terumo Glidewire Advantage (Terumo Medical Corp, Somerset, NJ, USA) provide a hydrophilic soft tip combined with a stiff but highly hydrophilic-coated 0.038-in shaft. This combination of relatively large wire, as opposed to angioplasty wire, tends to align the catheter more coaxially to transverse tortuous anatomy, while the hydrophilic tip encourages passage up the vessel. The shaft's coating interacts well with the artery despite modest straightening because of its nontraumatic nature. Similar to other hydrophilic wires, blind passage is not suggested and close observation of the path of the tip is required so as to not allow it to enter smaller vessels inadvertently. Using either a BAT approach or specialty wire can provide the operator with tools that can assist in a similar fashion in traversing challenging upper shoulder anatomy. Other techniques derived from telescopic catheter systems (child-in-mother techniques) or hydrophilic-coated catheter systems have also been suggested by other groups.[19,20] Although each technique has its advocates, the overriding

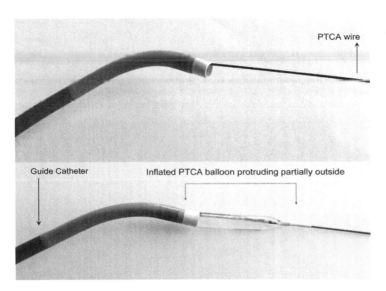

PTCA wire

Guide Catheter   Inflated PTCA balloon protruding partially outside

Fig. 2. Assembly for BAT technique.

principle is that the operator should have a logical plan for working through problems that are known to occur.

TRAVERSING THROUGH ARM AND CHEST VASCULATURE
Variant Anatomy of the Radial/Brachial Arteries
Identification and management of tortuosity
Tortuosity is more common in patients older than 70 years of age, long-standing diabetics, hypertensives, and women.[5–7,10,11,21–30] It is an important cause of resistance to the movement of a guidewire and/or a catheter. The RA angiogram reveals its severity and extent (**Fig. 4**). If the RA diameter is big, it is easy to negotiate the angiographic assembly through it. If the RA diameter is small and the tortuous segment is long, it should be crossed using a 0.025-in or 0.032-in J-shaped hydrophilic guidewire or a 0.014-in soft-tip PTCA guidewire. Carefully negotiate a catheter over the wire using a slow corkscrew movement under fluoroscopic guidance. Once the segment is crossed with the assembly, the procedure can be finished in the usual fashion. Direct push of the catheter is not recommended in this situation because it can induce reactive spasm. Spasm in a tortuous RA segment is a complex situation to manage. Repeat dosing of the spasmolytic cocktail may help working through a small caliber of RA and tortuous segment with or without spasm. The BAT technique should be reserved for most difficult situations.

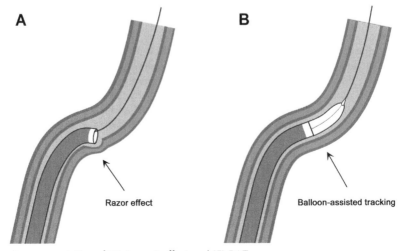

A

B

Razor effect

Balloon-assisted tracking

Fig. 3. Schematic representation of (A) "razor" effect and (B) BAT.

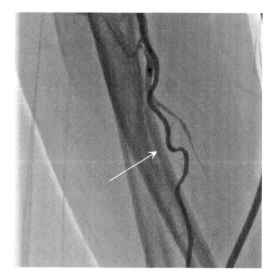

Fig. 4. RA tortuosity (*arrow*).

Identification and management of radial artery and brachial artery loops

Loops are another important form of anatomic variations to understand.[6–11,30] Normally, there is no resistance in advancement of guidewires and catheters up to the ascending aorta. Resistance in movement of a wire and/or a catheter is most commonly interpreted as RA spasm. Most times what initially appears as RA spasm is actually an anatomic variation in the form of tortuosity, loop, or curvature. A low threshold for performing an RA angiogram is critical because it defines the anatomy and helps define a working solution through a vast majority of these challenges.

Loops and curvatures are to be expected, and a radial operator needs to have a plan to work through this challenge. A consistent plan will reduce the apprehension of a new radialist and give additional confidence to an experienced operator. RA and BA loops can be simple or complex and can come in a variety of common and unique configurations, as shown in Figs. 5 and 6. When confronted with a loop, application of a logical course of action as described later has been helpful.

Steps in managing passage through radial artery and brachial artery loops
Define the task. When resistance is encountered in the movement of a wire and/or a catheter, inject diluted contrast to define the anatomy. If a simple loop is identified, one can work through it under fluoroscopic guidance. If it is a complex loop, multiple views should be taken (ie, right anterior oblique [RAO] and left anterior oblique [LAO], cranial or caudal angulations) (Fig. 7). Identify the view that best defines the loop. The view that is chosen can then be used as a "road map" for working through it.

Downsize the guidewire. If resistance is encountered in the passage of a standard 0.032-in or 0.035-in guidewire while working through the loop, remove the wire, because repeated attempts to negotiate it against the resistance can lead to perforation, spasm, and severe local pain (Fig. 8). A flexible guidewire (ie, 0.014-in soft-tip PTCA guidewire or a 0.025-in hydrophilic guidewire) should be used in place of a standard guidewire to cross the loop (Fig. 9). The tip of a guidewire (especially of a 0.014-in PTCA wire) can be shaped to the angle of the loop to facilitate crossing. When the guidewire crosses the loop, its tip is parked as high as possible (ie, high brachial, axillary, or subclavian region). Then, the catheter can be advanced over it. Sometimes, when these guidewires may not provide adequate support for the advancement of the catheters, the strategy should be changed.

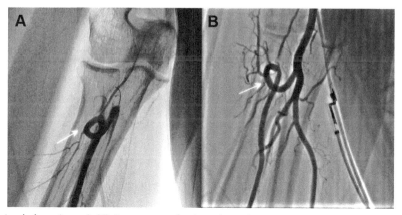

Fig. 5. (*A*) A simple loop (*arrow*). (*B*) A more complex loop (*arrow*).

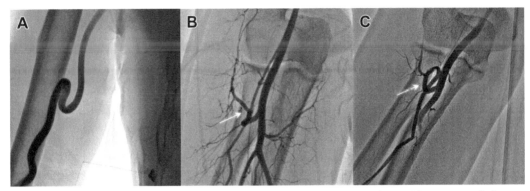

Fig. 6. (A) A double hairpin loop. (B) A radiocubital trunk (arrow). (C) A 360° loop with a very small diameter (arrow).

Use of buddy wires. When a single 0.014-in PTCA guidewire provides inadequate support for a catheter to cross the loop, the use of 1 or 2 additional guidewires should facilitate the advancement of the catheter by adding additional support (Fig. 10).

Straightening of the loop. Usually a catheter can easily negotiate over the wire and across a loop without disturbing the shape of the loop. Alternatively, if there is resistance in passage of the catheter while working through the loop, one can try pushing the catheter as far as possible into the loop, keeping the wire tip as high as possible (ie, in high brachial, axillary, or subclavian region). Then, pull the entire assembly slightly back (ie, the catheter along with guidewire). This maneuver opens up the loop and straightens it (Fig. 11). At this stage, advancement of the catheter across the loop becomes easy.

Exchanging the guidewire. This technique is helpful in addressing the most difficult loops. It can be used if the catheter is partly inside the loop, but has not crossed the entire loop and it is difficult to advance it any farther. Advance the catheter into the loop as far as possible. Exchange the thin guidewire for another guidewire to provide extra support. A 0.014-in PTCA guidewire can be exchanged with a 0.025-in hydrophilic guidewire and 0.025-in hydrophilic guidewire can be exchanged with a standard 0.035-in guidewire, if necessary (Fig. 12). Then, advance the catheter on the new wire. Avoid using a superstiff guidewire unless the loop has been crossed and the catheter tip is well into the higher segment (ie, high brachial, axillary, or subclavian region). This technique is useful in working through a difficult radiocubital trunk and a 360° loop with a very small diameter.

Use of balloon-assisted tracking. If a catheter cannot be negotiated through a complex 360° loop, BAT, which a high success rate, can be tried (Fig. 13). As the leading balloon is a PTCA device, an appropriately sized wire needs to be in place. The partially inflated balloon then acts as a bumper and wedge to permit catheter passage with reduced trauma.

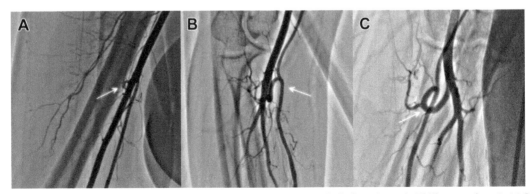

Fig. 7. (A) A hidden loop (arrow). (B) RA angiogram in RAO view revealed a loop (arrow). (C) The same loop in LAO view (arrow).

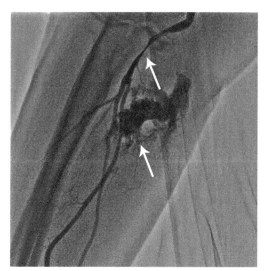

Fig. 8. A loop complicated by perforation and spasm (*arrow*).

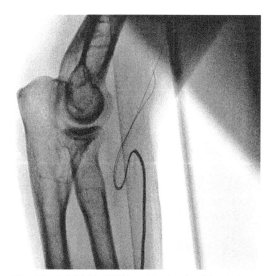

Fig. 10. A 0.014-in PTCA guidewire (buddy wire) was used to negotiate the loop.

Identification and management of anomalous origin of radial artery

This common anatomic variant is important to recognize. The caliber of RA in this situation is almost invariably small (Fig. 14).[6,9–11] High origins of the RA are an important cause of resistance to the movement of a catheter. It is commonly misinterpreted as an RA spasm. It may be suspected if the arterial course through the antecubital region appears somewhat more lateral than expected because the radial has not joined the brachial system. An RA angiogram reveals the diagnosis with a radial vessel clearly joining the brachial above the antecubital fossa. A very high originating radial may not be initially noticed on a short angiogram because the contrast may not have yet passed back down the BA, but this can be suspected if a definitive ulnar system cannot be seen on initial angiogram. Downsizing the catheter and repeat dosing of the spasmolytic cocktail help reduce the resistance in the passage of a catheter. The BAT technique can be very useful when the RA diameter is very small.[11,17] An algorithm for the management of loops is shown in Fig. 15.[6,11]

Acquired Abnormalities of the Radial/Brachial Arteries
Identification and management of atherosclerotic lesions

RA atherosclerosis is usually a part of the generalized atherosclerotic process.[6] It is possible to perform a diagnostic or interventional procedure successfully in this situation (Fig. 16). Atherosclerotic lesions in RA give resistance to the movement of a guidewire and/or a catheter. Once resistance is encountered, it is important to perform an RA angiogram.

If an RA angiogram reveals an atherosclerotic lesion, it is important to define its severity (mild to moderate or severe). If it is a mild obstruction, careful passage of the assembly through the affected segment under fluoroscopic guidance should allow the operator to perform and complete the procedure successfully. If it is a severe stenotic lesion, it is advisable to dilate the lesion with a PTCA catheter and then work through the affected segment. In both situations, a repeat dose of spasmolytic cocktail facilitates the passage of the assembly. The BAT technique should be reserved for difficult situations.

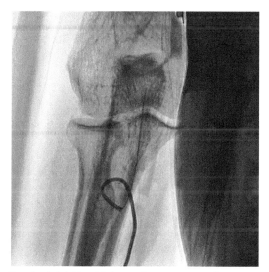

Fig. 9. A 0.014-in PTCA guidewire was used to negotiate the loop.

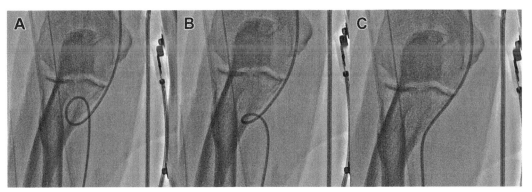

Fig. 11. (*A*) The catheter tip crossed the loop and entered the brachial artery. (*B*) To straighten the loop, the entire assembly was pulled back. (*C*) The loop was successfully straightened.

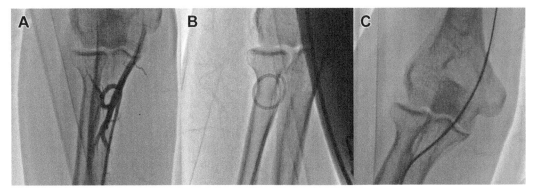

Fig. 12. (*A*) A 360° loop was negotiated using a 0.014-in soft-tip PTCA guidewire. (*B*) A 5-F pigtail catheter was deployed in the loop and the PTCA guidewire was removed. (*C*) A 0.035-in standard guidewire was negotiated across the loop; it was unfolded and the pigtail catheter was advanced farther.

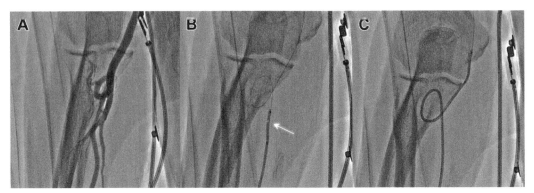

Fig. 13. (*A*) A 360° loop was profiled. (*B*) A 5F Optitorque TIG catheter was negotiated over a 0.014-in soft tip PTCA guide wire using BAT technique (*arrow*). (*C*) The catheter was successfully advanced through the loop without additional resistance. (*Courtesy of* [*B*] Terumo Interventional Systems, Somerset, NJ.)

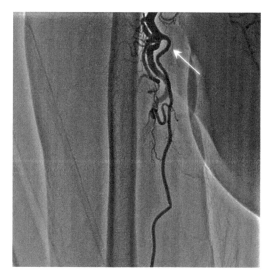

Fig. 14. Anomalous origin of the RA from the axillary artery (*arrow*).

Identification and management of calcification

Although uncommonly seen, it is important to identify this issue. Calcification can be patchy or diffuse.[6] Patchy calcification offers mild resistance to the passage of a guidewire and/or a catheter. However, it is easy to work through it using the standard technique. Diffuse calcification creates significant resistance to the passage of a guidewire and/or a catheter (Fig. 17). Instead of the standard push of the catheter over the wire, a slow corkscrew movement is recommended. This technique decreases the friction in the affected segment. Once the segment is crossed by the initial part of the catheter, the resistance disappears or decreases remarkably and rest of the diagnostic or interventional procedure can be completed in a regular fashion.

Subclavian and Innominate Tortuosities

SA and IA tortuosities can be the result of body changes from aging or inherent developmental variation from birth. They can be broadly classified as follows[12]:

1. Simple tortuosity: Angulation, usually greater than 90°, with minor calcification (Fig. 18A)
2. Complex tortuosity: Angulation less than 90° with hairpin, spiral, and other complex morphologies, with calcification, and/or atherosclerotic disease (see Fig. 18B, C)

Working through simple tortuosity

Resistance to the movement of a guidewire and/ or a catheter in the shoulder region should prompt consideration of this problem. Gentle

movement of assembly should bring successful entry into the ascending aorta. Normally, simple tortuosity does not create any challenges for a diagnostic or an interventional procedure. It is important to avoid a superstiff wire, unless the ascending or descending aorta has been entered, as it can create injury and dissection in this region. At times, deep inspiration facilitates the entry of guidewire and catheter in the ascending aorta. Although often overlooked when faced with adverse anatomy, this simple maneuver of taking a deep breath pulls the diaphragm down along with the thoracic contents, resulting in favorable change in the course of the vessel.

Working through complex tortuosity

The basic protocol is the same for working through complex tortuosity. However, at times, despite having a guidewire optimally positioned in ascending aorta, the catheter movement encounters severe resistance. At this stage, instead of pushing the catheter further over the wire, pulling it slightly back along with the guidewire straightens the tortuosity, allowing for smooth entry of a catheter in the ascending aorta. Usually a standard 0.032-in or a 0.035-in guidewire fails to enter ascending aorta and a 0.025-in or 0.032-in hydrophilic guidewire should be successful. At times, deep inspiration facilitates the entry of the guidewire and catheter in the ascending aorta. In the end, tortuosities are not necessarily reflected in the contralateral arm, and success may require a shift in access location without using the femoral artery.

Subclavian and Innominate Loops

A loop can be defined as a 360° turn of an artery in a subclavian and/or an innominate region. A loop can broadly be classified as follows[12]:

1. Simple loop: A 360° large-diameter turn of an artery (Fig. 19A)
2. Complex loop: A 360° small-diameter turn of an artery (see Fig. 19B)

Working through a simple loop

This loop most commonly exists at an innominate-aortic arch junction; however, it can happen anywhere in the course of the subclavian-innominate region. It is usually possible to traverse through a simple loop using a standard 0.032-in or 0.035-in guidewire. If an operator encounters significant resistance, a 0.025-in or a 0.032-in hydrophilic guidewire may help to traverse complete course of the loop to enter ascending aorta. If that technique fails, a soft-tipped 0.014-in PTCA guidewire is negotiated carefully, under fluoroscopic

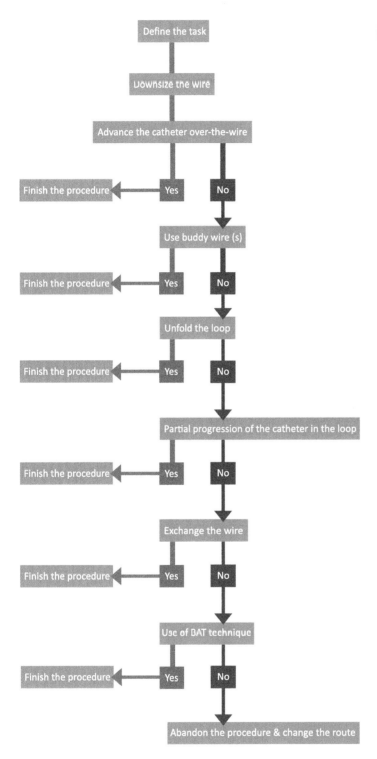

Fig. 15. Management of RA and BA loops.

guidance, to enter the ascending aorta. If a diagnostic or a guide catheter also encounters severe resistance at the site of loop over a PTCA wire, use of the BAT technique predictably brings success for ascending aortic entry.

Working through a complex loop
The basic protocol for working through a complex loop remains the same as working through a simple loop. However, with this situation, most

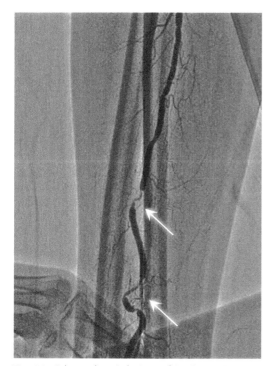

Fig. 16. Atherosclerotic lesions of RA (*arrows*).

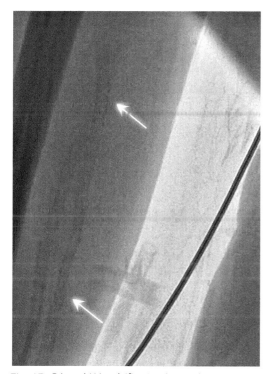

Fig. 17. RA and UA calcification (*arrows*).

of the time only the BAT technique predictably brings success for the ascending aortic entry.

Subclavian and Innominate Stenosis
Working through subclavian and innominate stenosis

Working through subclavian and innominate stenosis is an uncommon issue that, when it occurs, is of atherosclerotic origin. Whenever resistance is encountered with the movement of a standard 0.032-in or a 0.035-in guidewire and/or a catheter, this problem should be suspected. A hand injection with contrast in this region establishes the diagnosis (Fig. 20). At times, more than one view in different angulations may be required to define the diagnosis. Once the diagnosis is made, a 0.025-in or a 0.032-in hydrophilic guidewire is used to cross the stenosis for ascending or descending aortic entry. At times, using a soft-tipped 0.014-in PTCA guidewire may bring success. Once the stenosis is crossed with the guidewire, a diagnostic or a guide catheter can be negotiated carefully through it under fluoroscopic guidance to enter ascending or descending aorta for completion of a coronary or a peripheral procedure. In case of a severe and complex stenosis, the BAT technique helps the catheter enter into the ascending aorta. It is important to use fluoroscopic guidance while working through this region to prevent damage to the carotid, vertebral, or internal mammary artery ostia.[12] Most subtotal subclavian-innominate stenoses can be treated with balloon angioplasty and stenting at the same time or as a staged procedure later on. If a total subclavian or innominate stenosis is encountered, switching to the other RA or even the femoral approach should be considered. A feeble or absent radial pulse gives a clue for this diagnosis.[12] However, in most instances, the radial pulse is normal with a normal Allen test because of the development of extensive collaterals.

Arteria Lusoria (Retro-Esophageal Subclavian)

Congenital abnormalities of the upper extremity vasculature are relatively rare, but are best represented by the retro-esophageal SA as known as arteria lusoria. Arteria lusoria is the most common congenital aberrancy of the right SA characterized topographically as follows: the artery originates distal to the left SA as the fourth main branch of the aortic arch and turns to the right behind the esophagus, in front of vertebral column (Fig. 21). The incidence in the literature varies from 0.2% to 1.7%.[6,9,10,12,31] In about 60% of cases, the right subclavian originates from an outpouch or defect in the aorta known as a Kommerell diverticulum

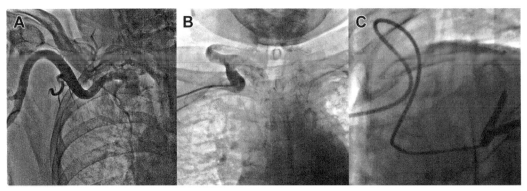

Fig. 18. (*A*) An example of simple subclavian tortuosity. (*B*) An example of complex subclavian tortuosity. (*C*) Successful left coronary artery (LCA) cannulation using a 5-F Optitorque TIG catheter. (*Courtesy of* Terumo Interventional Systems, Somerset, NJ.)

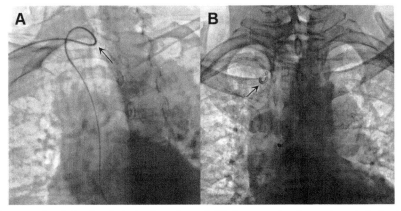

Fig. 19. (*A*) An example of simple subclavian loop (*arrow*). (*B*) An example of complex subclavian loop (*arrow*).

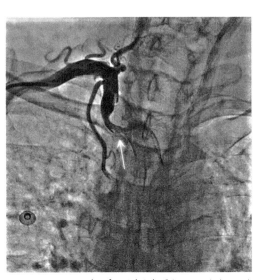

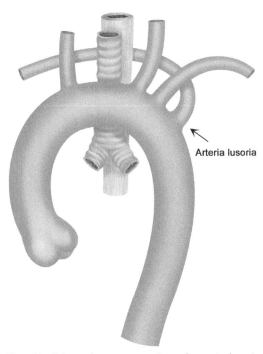

Fig. 20. An example of ostial right SA stenosis (*arrow*).

Fig. 21. Schematic representation of arteria lusoria (*arrow*).

that can result in localized aneurysm formation.[32,33] The right carotid artery arises directly from the arch, as a first major branch of aortic arch.

Working through arteria lusoria

The protocol for working through the arteria lusoria is divided into 2 parts[6,12]:

1. Entering the ascending aorta through arteria lusoria
2. Cannulation of coronary arteries.

Entering the ascending aorta through arteria lusoria

It is important to work in the 40° LAO view.

Step 1: The catheter and guidewire have a tendency to enter the descending aorta. Repeated entry in the descending aorta despite using the usual technique should prompt an operator to suspect arteria lusoria. If this happens, withdraw the catheter and guidewire together as an assembly. After asking the patient to take a deep breath, gently push the 0.035-in standard guidewire. If it enters the ascending aorta effortlessly, negotiate the catheter over the guidewire into the ascending aorta (Fig. 22).

Step 2: If step 1 is not successful, keep the guidewire in the descending aorta. Remove the first catheter tried. Take a 5-F internal mammary artery (IMA) diagnostic catheter and put it into the descending aorta over the guidewire. Then, try the step 1 maneuver. In many cases, this approach will be successful for entry into the ascending aorta.

Step 3: If the IMA catheter fails, a 5-F Simmons-1 catheter can be used to enter the ascending aorta.

Step 4: If the 0.035-in standard guidewire has a tendency to slip into the descending aorta, the second choices are a 0.032-in or a 0.025-in hydrophilic guidewire. The slippery characteristic of a hydrophilic guidewire facilitates entry into the ascending aorta even through challenging anatomy.

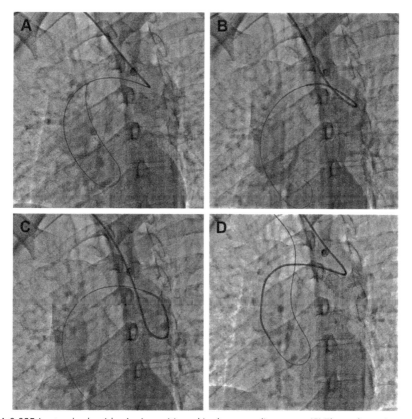

Fig. 22. (A) A 0.035-in standard guidewire is positioned in the ascending aorta. (B) The catheter is negotiated over the wire to enter the ascending aorta. (C) Although the catheter is pushed over the wire, it has a tendency to enter the descending aorta, along with the guidewire loop. (D) The whole assembly is gently pulled back, and the catheter is slowly pushed over the wire to enter the ascending aorta.

Cannulation of coronary arteries.   Once the guidewire and the catheter are in the ascending aorta, the following steps are to be observed for cannulation of coronary ostia.

> Step 1: Remove the standard 0.035-in guidewire or the hydrophilic guidewire, keeping the catheter in the ascending aorta.
> Step 2: Use a 0.035-in superstiff guidewire and make a loop of wire in the ascending aorta. Slowly negotiate the catheter over it so that the assembly (catheter and guidewire) can traverse the aortic loop.
> Step 3: Slowly pull the guidewire slightly inside the mouth of the catheter and pull the assembly back. This maneuver usually cannulates the left coronary artery. For cannulation of the right coronary artery, a slow and gentle clockwise rotation of the assembly is done.

For diagnostic procedures, use an Optitorque TIG, a Judkins left, or an Amplatz left catheter to cannulate the left coronary ostium. Sometimes, a 5-F extra backup (EBU) guide catheter is useful for cannulating the left coronary ostium. For cannulating the right coronary ostium, a Judkins right, an Amplatz right, or an Amplatz left curve can be used (Fig. 23).

For intervention in the left coronary system, choose an EBU guide catheter as a first choice. If this is not successful, use of an Amplatz left or a wider Judkins left curve may help. For intervention in the right coronary system, an Amplatz right catheter is the first choice. If this does not succeed, a Judkins right or an Amplatz left catheter can be used (Fig. 24).

At any stage during cannulation of the coronary ostium, do not push too much or the assembly may flip into the descending aorta.

The steps may seem complicated, but arteria lusoria is very rare, and patience and perseverance can help complete the procedure in the usual fashion. Although beginners should opt for an alternative approach in patients with known arteria lusoria, most cases are first recognized at the time of catheterization. If the first few

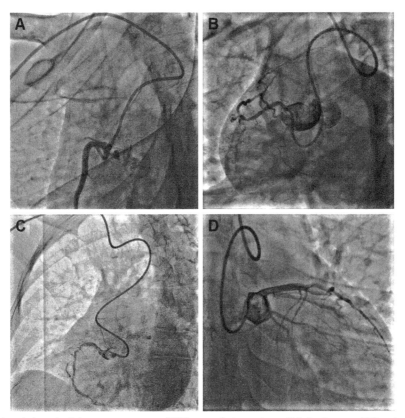

Fig. 23. (A) Arteria lusoria-right coronary artery (RCA) cannulation using a 5-F Optitorque TIG catheter (Terumo, Japan). (B) Arteria lusoria-RCA cannulation using a 5-F AL1 diagnostic catheter. (C) Arteria lusoria-diagnostic RCA cannulation using a 5-F EBU guide catheter. (D) Arteria lusoria-LCA cannulation using a 5-F AL1 diagnostic catheter. (Courtesy of [A] Terumo Interventional Systems, Somerset, NJ.)

attempts to enter the ascending aorta are unsuccessful, gracefully switch to left radial or the femoral route. Although there is always the operator's pride at risk, consideration of extra contrast and radiation requirements to finish the procedure and the knowledge that there may be an associated aneurysm at risk for rupture should temper the operator's persistence.

With experience, the failure rate of working through arteria lusoria can be significantly minimized.

Combined Challenges in Subclavian and Innominate Region

The combined challenges in the subclavian and innominate region can be broadly classified as follows[12]:

1. Tortuosity with loop: In this case, a complex subclavian tortuosity with loop has been successfully traversed and both coronaries have been cannulated (Fig. 25).

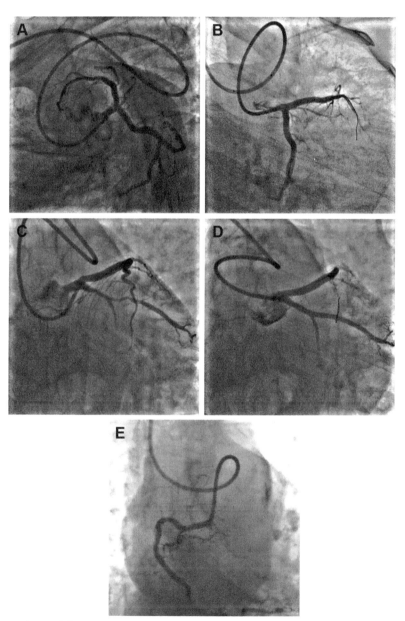

Fig. 24. (A) Arteria lusoria-left anterior descending artery (LAD) intervention using a 6-F EBU guide catheter. (B) Arteria lusoria-LAD intervention in progress using a 5-F EBU guide catheter. (C) Arteria lusoria-LCA cannulation was done using a 6-F EBU guide catheter. (D) Arteria lusoria-left circumflex artery (LCX) intervention was successfully completed using a 6-F EBU guide catheter. (E) Arteria lusoria-RCA intervention was successfully completed using a 6-F JR4 guide catheter.

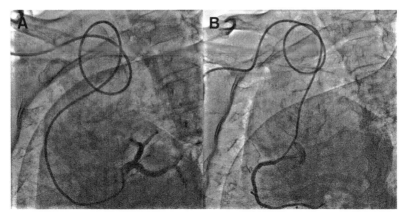

Fig. 25. (A) A complex subclavian tortuosity combined with a complex loop was crossed and the LCA was cannulated using a 5-F Optitorque TIG catheter. (B) The RCA was cannulated using the same catheter. (*Courtesy of* [A] Terumo Interventional Systems, Somerset, NJ.)

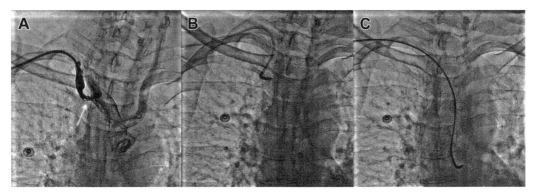

Fig. 26. (A) Subclavian tortuosity with tight stenosis (*arrow*). (B) Use of the BAT technique. (C) Successful catheter entry into the ascending aorta.

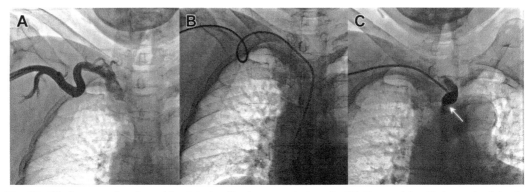

Fig. 27. (A) An example of combined tortuosity, loop, and stenosis. (B) Successful catheter entry into the ascending aorta. (C) A tight innominate stenosis is revealed (*arrow*).

2. Tortuosity with stenosis: In this case, the BAT technique was used to traverse a tortuosity associated with a severe stenosis (Fig. 26).
3. Tortuosity with loop and stenosis: In this case, a catheter on a 0.025-in hydrophilic guidewire successfully crossed a complex tortuosity associated with loop and a critical stenosis (Fig. 27).
4. Tortuosity with arteria lusoria: In this case, a catheter on a 0.032-in hydrophilic guidewire successfully crossed a complex tortuosity and arteria lusoria (Fig. 28).

Working through combined challenges
Whenever an operator encounters resistance with a guidewire and/or a catheter movement in this region, it is important to document the problem by injecting the contrast. If there are more complex issues, the operator may require injections in several views to document the anatomic challenges. Once any of these combined challenges is identified, the operator should use the protocols described to work through them in a judicious manner. In most cases, these challenges can be overcome; however, in rare situations it may be wise to abandon the procedure and change the route if the ascending aortic entry is not possible. Even the most experienced operators will occasionally be unable to overcome a particular vascular challenge. The initial access site switchover to the contralateral radial or femoral approach should be considered not only to prevent harm to the patient from excessive procedural time and exposure to contrast and radiation, but also to prevent harm to the operator and staff.

SUMMARY

Management of the most important vascular challenges for transradial procedures can be accomplished following simple algorithms. Such approaches should increase the comfort level of an operator for successful completion of a TRA procedure. However, an operator may rarely encounter difficulty in tracking a catheter or a guidewire despite applying all the techniques including BAT. It is important to switch over to either the contralateral radial or the femoral approach to facilitate procedure completion. By incrementally advancing the vascular skill of operators using the radial approach, basic radial operators can evolve into advanced operators capable of more fully providing transradial services and therefore improving their patients' outcomes.

ACKNOWLEDGMENTS

The authors are grateful to Mr Yash Soni for his extremely valuable support during the preparation of this article.

REFERENCES

1. Campeau L. Percutaneous radial artery approach for coronary angiography. Cathet Cardiovasc Diagn 1989;16:3–7.
2. Kiemeneij F, Laarman GJ. Transradial artery Palmaz-Schatz coronary stent implantation: results of a single-center feasibility study. Am Heart J 1995;130.14–21.
3. Kiemeneij F, Laarman GJ, de Melker E. Transradial artery coronary angioplasty. Am Heart J 1995;129: 1–7.
4. Lotan C, Hasin Y, Mosseri M, et al. Transradial approach for coronary angiography and angioplasty. Am J Cardiol 1995;76:164–7.
5. Rao SV, Ou FS, Wang TY, et al. Trends in the prevalence and outcomes of radial and femoral approaches to percutaneous coronary intervention: a report from the National Cardiovascular Data Registry. JACC Cardiovasc Interv 2008;1(4):379–86.
6. Patel T, Shah S, Pancholy S. Patel's atlas of transradial intervention: the basics & beyond. Malvern (PA): HMP Communications; 2012.
7. Barbeau G. Radial loop and extreme vessel tortuosity in the transradial approach: advantage of hydrophilic-coated guidewires and catheters. Catheter Cardiovasc Interv 2003;59(4):442–50.

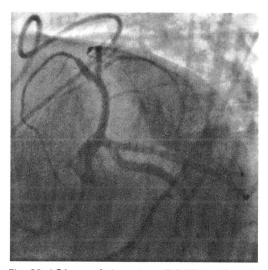

Fig. 28. LCA cannulation using a 5-F EBU guide catheter through a complex subclavian tortuosity associated with arteria lusoria in the LAO caudal view.

8. Bazemore E, Mann T. Problems and complications of the transradial approach for coronary interventions: a review. J Invasive Cardiol 2005;17(3):156–9.

9. Valsecchi O, Vassileva A, Musumeci G, et al. Failure of transradial approach during coronary interventions: anatomic considerations. Catheter Cardiovasc Interv 2006;67(6):870–8.

10. Dehghani P, Mohammad A, Bajaj R, et al. Mechanism and predictors of failed transradial approach for percutaneous coronary interventions. JACC Cardiovasc Interv 2009;2(11):1057–64.

11. Patel T, Shah S, Pancholy S, et al. Working through complexities of radial and brachial vasculature during transradial approach. Catheter Cardiovasc Interv 2014;83(7):1074–88.

12. Patel T, Shah S, Pancholy S, et al. Working through challenges of subclavian, innominate, and aortic arch regions during transradial approach. Catheter Cardiovasc Interv 2014;84(2):224–35.

13. Lo TS, Nolan J, Fountzopoulos E, et al. Radial artery anomaly and its influence on transradial coronary procedural outcome. Heart 2009;95:410–5.

14. Rodríguez-Niedenführ M, Vázquez T, Nearn L, et al. Variations of the arterial pattern in the upper limb revisited: a morphological and statistical study, with a review of the literature. J Anat 2001; 199(Pt 5):547–66.

15. Kern MJ. Letter to editor: unusual radial artery calcification. Catheter Cardiovasc Interv 2013; 82(5):853.

16. Nanto S, Ohara T, Shimonagata T, et al. A technique for changing a PTCA balloon catheter over regular-length guidewire. Cathet Cardiovasc Diagn 1994;32:274–7.

17. Patel T, Shah S, Pancholy S. Balloon-assisted tracking: a must-know technique to overcome difficult anatomy during transradial approach. Catheter Cardiovasc Interv 2014;83(2):211–20.

18. Pancholy S, Coppola J, Patel T. Subcutaneous administration of nitroglycerin to facilitate radial artery cannulation. Catheter Cardiovasc Interv 2006; 68(3):389–91.

19. Hayashida K, Louvard Y, Lefevre T. Transradial complex coronary interventions using a five-in-six system. Catheter Cardiovasc Interv 2011;77(1):63–8.

20. Tomassini F, Gagnor A, Varbella F. Successful use of an extra-long hydrophilic-coated sheath in enlarged aorta to overcome extreme tortuosity of right subclavian artery. J Invasive Cardiol 2011;23:E56–8.

21. Caputo RP, Tremmel JA, Rao S, et al. Transradial arterial access for coronary and peripheral procedures: executive summary by the transradial committee of the SCAI. Catheter Cardiovasc Interv 2011;78(6):823–39.

22. Kiemeneij F, Laarman GJ, Odekerken D, et al. A randomized comparison of percutaneous transluminal coronary angioplasty by the radial, brachial and femoral approaches: the access study. J Am Coll Cardiol 1997;29(6):1269–75.

23. Agostoni P, Biondi-Zoccai GG, de Benedictis ML, et al. Radial versus femoral approach for percutaneous coronary diagnostic and interventional procedures; Systematic overview and meta-analysis of randomized trials. J Am Coll Cardiol 2004;44:349–56.

24. Jolly SS, Amlani S, Hamon M, et al. Radial versus femoral access for coronary angiography or intervention and the impact on major bleeding and ischemic events: a systematic review and meta-analysis of randomized trials. Am Heart J 2009; 157(1):131–40.

25. Bertrand O, Rao S, Pancholy S, et al. Transradial approach for coronary angiography and interventions: results of the first international transradial practice survey. JACC Cardiovasc Interv 2010; 3(10):1032–4.

26. Gilchrist I. Transradial catheterization's grass roots epidemic. JACC Cardiovasc Interv 2010;3(10): 1032–4.

27. Ho P. Transradial complex coronary interventions: expanding the comfort zone. J Invasive Cardiol 2008;20(5):222.

28. Amoroso G, Kiemeneij F. Transradial access for primary percutaneous coronary intervention: the next standard of care? Heart 2010;96(17):1341–4.

29. Patel T, Shah S, Sanghavi K, et al. Management of radial and brachial artery perforations during transradial procedures – a practical approach. J Invasive Cardiol 2009;21(10):544–7.

30. Gilchrist I. Transradial technical tips. Catheter Cardiovasc Interv 2000;49(3):353–4.

31. Abhaichand R, Louvard Y, Gobeil J, et al. The problem of arteria lusoria in right transradial coronary angiography and angioplasty. Catheter Cardiovasc Interv 2001;54(2):196–201.

32. Kommere LB. Verlagerung des Oesophagus durch eine abnorm verlaufende Arteria subclavia dextra (Arteria lusoria). Fortschr Geb Röntgenstr 1936;54: 590–5.

33. Felson B. Ruptured anomalous right subclavian artery: aneurysm or diverticulum? Semin Roentgenol 1989;24(2):121–6.

Diagnostic and Guide Catheter Selection and Manipulation for Radial Approach

CrossMark

Carlos E. Alfonso, MD, Mauricio G. Cohen, MD, FACC, FSCAI*

KEYWORDS

- Transradial angiography • Transradial percutaneous coronary intervention • Cardiac catheterization • Coronary angiography

KEY POINTS

- Mechanisms and predictors of transradial (TR) failure include arterial spasm, anatomic limitations, failure to cannulate the target vessel, and inadequate guide support.
- Adequate guide catheter support is key for successful TR percutaneous coronary intervention.
- Finesse and careful maneuvering and torquing are important for catheter manipulation and coronary engagement; the operator should never push against resistance.
- Guide catheter selection should depend on the operator's comfort level and expertise.
- A "single-catheter strategy" is feasible and may be beneficial in certain scenarios.

INTRODUCTION

The multiple advantages of transradial (TR) catheterization and percutaneous coronary interventions (PCI) have been enumerated in the past and include reduced bleeding risk; a trend toward decrease in ischemic end points of death, stroke, or myocardial infarction; reduced length of stay and costs; early ambulation; and improved patient comfort for most patients.[1,2]

The current success rate with TR PCI is greater than 90%, which is similar to that of transfemoral (TF) PCI. When the success rate of TR versus TF PCI was compared in a systematic review and meta-analysis of 23 randomized trials with 7020 patients, there was a nonsignificant trend for an increased incidence of inability to cross lesions with TR access compared with the TF approach (3.4% vs 4.7%; $P = .21$).[3] There was

also a trend toward increased procedural failure, and a significant difference in the need for access site crossover (odds ratio, 3.82 [2.83–5.15]).[3] A single-center study examined the mechanism of TR PCI procedural failure in 2100 TR PCI procedures ($\leq$6F catheter) performed by low- to intermediate-volume operators. Procedural failure occurred in 98 (4.7%) patients. Mechanisms and predictors of TR PCI procedural failure included inability to puncture the radial artery, arterial spasm, anatomic limitations, failure to cannulate the target vessel, and inadequate guide support (Fig. 1).[4] To further improve success rates with TR catheterization and PCI, it is important to address each of these obstacles. About one-third of failures to complete TR PCI were caused by lack of guiding catheter support either because of subclavian tortuosity or inadequate backup support.

M.G. Cohen is a Consultant for Accumed, Terumo Medical, and Merit Medical. He is on the Speakers' Bureau for Medtronic. C.E. Alfonso has nothing to disclose.

Cardiac Catheterization Laboratory, Cardiovascular Division, Department of Medicine, University of Miami Hospital, University of Miami Miller School of Medicine, 1400 Northwest 12th Avenue, Miami, FL 33136, USA

* Corresponding author. University of Miami Hospital, 1400 Northwest 12th Avenue, Suite 1179, Miami, FL 33136.
E-mail address: mgcohen@med.miami.edu

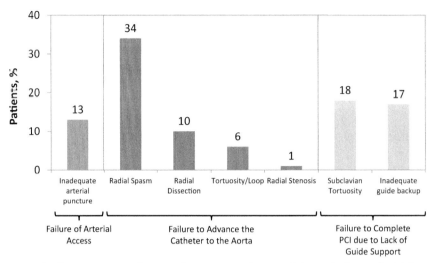

Fig. 1. Failure modes for TR PCI. Data from nearly 100 cases of TR PCI failure, which stratified failure into either failure of arterial access, failure to navigate to ascending aorta, or failure of guide support and their subcategories as shown. (*Data from* Dehghani P, Mohammad A, Bajaj R, et al. Mechanism and predictors of failed transradial approach for percutaneous coronary interventions. JACC Cardiovasc Interv 2009;2:1057–64.)

Guiding catheter selection, use, and engagement are essential factors for coronary interventions in general, but it is compulsory for TR PCI. Although some disadvantages are noted, most of these can be overcome with further refinement of techniques and use of certain tips and tricks. This article reviews some of the essentials for guide catheter selection, navigation of the anatomy, and manipulation during TR catheterization and PCI.

TRANSRADIAL CATHETERIZATION AND INTERVENTION

The general tenets of cardiac catheterization and PCI remain the same either with TR or TF access. However, TR catheterization and interventions require the acquisition of various additional skill sets including radial arterial puncture, the ability to navigate the upper extremity vasculature with full understanding of anatomic variations, and catheter selection and coronary engagement technique.

NAVIGATING THE AORTIC ARCH AND GREAT VESSELS

In most cases, accessing the ascending aorta via the right or left radial artery does not pose major challenges. In some cases, however, the degree of tortuosity within the great vessels, the anatomic variations, and the take-off angle of the great vessels from the aortic arch can make navigation of the arch more challenging

(Fig. 2). Although potentially a nuisance, it is still possible to navigate through most of these anatomic variations and safely proceed with TR PCI. Practical tips for navigating the upper extremity vasculature and engaging the coronary arteries are presented in Box 1. Certain anatomic variants, such as arteria lusoria

| Box 1 |
| Practical tips for guide catheter navigation and coronary engagement |
| *Advancing guiding catheter to ascending aorta* |
| Perform catheter exchanges with the tip of a 260-cm long wire in the aortic root |
| Stiff wires can be used in severe cases of tortuosity for additional support |
| If needed, use hydrophilic wires to navigate tortuous subclavian anatomy |
| Have patient take deep inspiration to help navigate and straighten tortuosity |
| If not sure of wire position, perform a limited angiogram to understand anatomy |
| *Engaging coronary artery* |
| Advance catheter and start manipulation over the wire deep into aortic cusp of interest |
| To prevent knotting and kinking, keep wire within the guide catheter during manipulations |
| Once the catheter is engaged in the coronary ostium, pull back gently to improve coaxiality and avoid dissections |

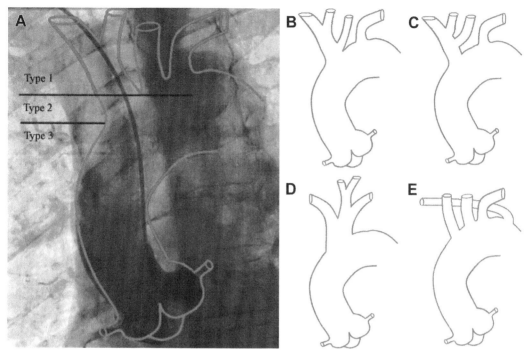

Fig. 2. Aortic arch anatomy variations. The aortic arch can be characterized into three types based on the vertical distance from the origin of the innominate artery to the top of the arch (*A*). A type 1 arch has a distance that is less than one times the diameter of the left common carotid artery (CCA). A type 2 arch originates from one to two CCA diameters from the top of the arch, and a type 3 arch originates more than two CCA diameters from the top of the arch. In addition, some variation in the take-offs of the great vessels can be observed, including variants where the left carotid originates from the innominate artery trunk (*B–C*), a true bovine arch (*D*), and arteria lusoria (*E*).

(see Fig. 2E), although uncommon, may make this practically impossible and may necessitate crossover to a left radial or femoral approach.[5]

For coronary engagement, finesse is required rather than force. Active catheter holding is recommended because there may be multiple friction points in the subclavian and the aorta. Small (finger-based) clockwise and counterclockwise torquing movements are suggested. Extensive torquing and manipulation can cause catheter kinking and knotting.

DIAGNOSTIC CATHETER SELECTION AND MANIPULATION

Femoral catheter shapes, such as the Judkins family of catheters, perform adequately from the left or right radial approach and hence allow femoral operators to avoid major changes in catheter selection or manipulation during their learning curve. When using traditional Judkins-shaped catheters, it may be necessary to use a catheter with a shorter secondary curve (Judkins left [JL] 3.5 instead of JL4) for the left coronary system. To engage the left coronary artery

(LCA) with the JL3.5 catheter certain simple maneuvers are followed (Fig. 3).

- Leaving the 0.035-in guidewire inside the catheter (but not protruding) prevents the catheter from curling up during manipulation.
- The JL catheter is gently torqued clockwise as it navigates through the ascending aorta pointing toward the left coronary cusp.
- When close to the left coronary ostium, final torquing movements usually allow for selective cannulation.
- If the catheter tip points below the ostium, advancing the catheter gently prolapses the secondary curve of the catheter into the sinus of Valsalva and points the tip up toward the ostium.
- Once engaged, a slight catheter pull back with gentle clockwise torque allows for more coaxial engagement.

To engage the right coronary artery (RCA), it may be necessary to increase by 1 cm the right Judkins curve, so instead of a Judkins right (JR)

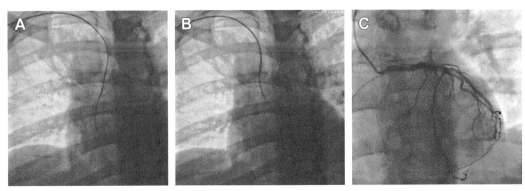

Fig. 3. Left coronary artery cannulation with a Judkins left catheter is performed easily by advancing the catheter over the wire to the aortic cusp (*A*). When the catheter is pulled back with slight clockwise or counterclockwise rotation, it pulls into the left coronary ostium (*B*). Slight manipulation allows for coaxial engagement (*C*).

4, use a JR5; however, a JR4 still remains the most commonly used catheter. Catheter manipulation for RCA engagement is similar to the femoral approach. The JR catheter is advanced into the right coronary cusp and then pulled back while torquing clockwise until the catheter finds the ostium of the RCA.

A "single-catheter" approach where one catheter is used to engage both coronary ostia is possible with various catheter shapes and has various benefits (Fig. 4). A decrease in catheter exchanges and manipulation reduces the occurrence of vasospasm and therefore increases patient comfort.[6] A single-catheter strategy may lead to further reduction in procedure and fluoroscopy time, radiation exposure, and use of fewer catheters compared with the Judkins catheter technique. One drawback to a single-catheter strategy remains the ability to engage both coronary ostia completely coaxially

every time. Various catheter shapes have now been designed that allow for the single-catheter strategy and include the Kimny, Tiger, Jacky, and Ikari catheters. The Tiger (Optitorque Terumo, Somerset, NJ) is a double-braided catheter with a flat segment in the third portion of the loop, which provides contralateral backup support, and a side hole just proximal to the tip. Engagement of the LCA with the Tiger or Jacky (Optitorque Terumo) catheter is somewhat similar to the engagement with the JL and is performed as follows (see Fig. 4; Fig. 5):

- Keep the 0.035-in wire within the catheter.
- Place the tip of the catheter just below the LCA and facing left.
- Pull back the wire slowly, making the tip of the catheter point upward to engage the left main coronary ostium.

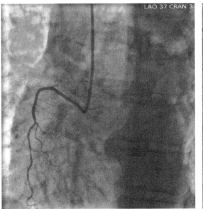
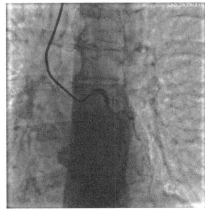

Fig. 4. LCA and RCA cannulation with a single-catheter strategy using a Tiger catheter. After engagement of the LCA as described, gently pulling back and applying clockwise rotation on the catheter allows the same catheter to engage and complete angiography of the RCA.

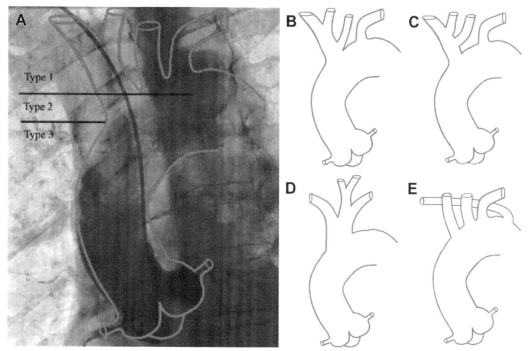

Fig. 2. Aortic arch anatomy variations. The aortic arch can be characterized into three types based on the vertical distance from the origin of the innominate artery to the top of the arch (*A*). A type 1 arch has a distance that is less than one times the diameter of the left common carotid artery (CCA). A type 2 arch originates from one to two CCA diameters from the top of the arch, and a type 3 arch originates more than two CCA diameters from the top of the arch. In addition, some variation in the take-offs of the great vessels can be observed, including variants where the left carotid originates from the innominate artery trunk (*B–C*), a true bovine arch (*D*), and arteria lusoria (*E*).

(see Fig. 2E), although uncommon, may make this practically impossible and may necessitate crossover to a left radial or femoral approach.[5]

For coronary engagement, finesse is required rather than force. Active catheter holding is recommended because there may be multiple friction points in the subclavian and the aorta. Small (finger-based) clockwise and counterclockwise torquing movements are suggested. Extensive torquing and manipulation can cause catheter kinking and knotting.

DIAGNOSTIC CATHETER SELECTION AND MANIPULATION

Femoral catheter shapes, such as the Judkins family of catheters, perform adequately from the left or right radial approach and hence allow femoral operators to avoid major changes in catheter selection or manipulation during their learning curve. When using traditional Judkins-shaped catheters, it may be necessary to use a catheter with a shorter secondary curve (Judkins left [JL] 3.5 instead of JL4) for the left coronary system. To engage the left coronary artery

(LCA) with the JL3.5 catheter certain simple maneuvers are followed (Fig. 3).

- Leaving the 0.035-in guidewire inside the catheter (but not protruding) prevents the catheter from curling up during manipulation.
- The JL catheter is gently torqued clockwise as it navigates through the ascending aorta pointing toward the left coronary cusp.
- When close to the left coronary ostium, final torquing movements usually allow for selective cannulation.
- If the catheter tip points below the ostium, advancing the catheter gently prolapses the secondary curve of the catheter into the sinus of Valsalva and points the tip up toward the ostium.
- Once engaged, a slight catheter pull back with gentle clockwise torque allows for more coaxial engagement.

To engage the right coronary artery (RCA), it may be necessary to increase by 1 cm the right Judkins curve, so instead of a Judkins right (JR)

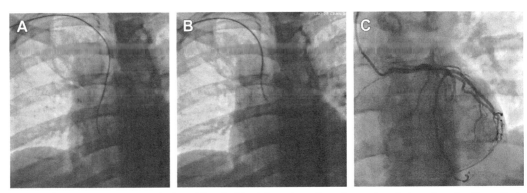

Fig. 3. Left coronary artery cannulation with a Judkins left catheter is performed easily by advancing the catheter over the wire to the aortic cusp (A). When the catheter is pulled back with slight clockwise or counterclockwise rotation, it pulls into the left coronary ostium (B). Slight manipulation allows for coaxial engagement (C).

4, use a JR5; however, a JR4 still remains the most commonly used catheter. Catheter manipulation for RCA engagement is similar to the femoral approach. The JR catheter is advanced into the right coronary cusp and then pulled back while torquing clockwise until the catheter finds the ostium of the RCA.

A "single-catheter" approach where one catheter is used to engage both coronary ostia is possible with various catheter shapes and has various benefits (Fig. 4). A decrease in catheter exchanges and manipulation reduces the occurrence of vasospasm and therefore increases patient comfort.[6] A single-catheter strategy may lead to further reduction in procedure and fluoroscopy time, radiation exposure, and use of fewer catheters compared with the Judkins catheter technique. One drawback to a single-catheter strategy remains the ability to engage both coronary ostia completely coaxially

every time. Various catheter shapes have now been designed that allow for the single-catheter strategy and include the Kimny, Tiger, Jacky, and Ikari catheters. The Tiger (Optitorque Terumo, Somerset, NJ) is a double-braided catheter with a flat segment in the third portion of the loop, which provides contralateral backup support, and a side hole just proximal to the tip. Engagement of the LCA with the Tiger or Jacky (Optitorque Terumo) catheter is somewhat similar to the engagement with the JL and is performed as follows (see Fig. 4; Fig. 5):

- Keep the 0.035-in wire within the catheter.
- Place the tip of the catheter just below the LCA and facing left.
- Pull back the wire slowly, making the tip of the catheter point upward to engage the left main coronary ostium.

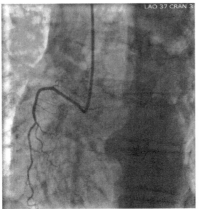
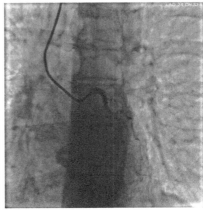

Fig. 4. LCA and RCA cannulation with a single-catheter strategy using a Tiger catheter. After engagement of the LCA as described, gently pulling back and applying clockwise rotation on the catheter allows the same catheter to engage and complete angiography of the RCA.

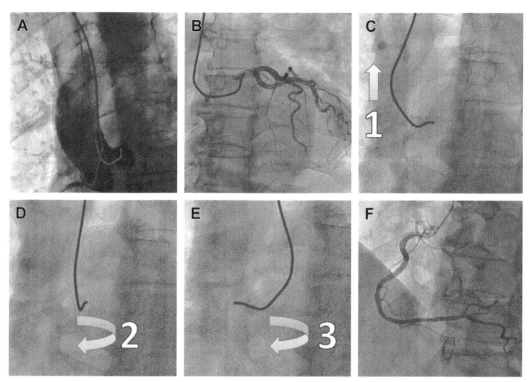

Fig. 5. Left and right coronary artery cannulation with a single-catheter strategy using a Jacky catheter. The catheter position for engagement of both the left and right coronary ostium is shown (A). Changing from the left coronary artery (B) to the right coronary artery can be performed by first disengaging the catheter by pulling back slightly (C), then clockwise rotation (D, E) allows for engagement of the right coronary artery, and some slight advancement allows for coaxial catheter engagement before right coronary angiography (F).

- Slight clockwise or counterclockwise torque can be applied for more selective and coaxial cannulation.
- Engaging the RCA is performed by applying clockwise motion until the tip enters the right sinus of Valsalva and eventually engages the RCA.

Arterial pressure at the catheter tip should be carefully monitored during manipulation because the catheter has a tendency to selectively engage the conus branch. The Tiger catheter can be used to successfully cannulate the LCA and RCA in a high proportion of cases.[7,8]

During TR catheterization, torque usually stores with manipulation and catheters have a tendency to easily disengage from the coronary ostia. To prevent this, careful attention is needed not to excessively force contrast injection, and to preserve position maintaining constant control of the catheter at the hub.

Alternatively to the universal catheters, the JL3.5 catheter can also be used to engage the RCA, because it assumes a shape similar to that of a JR4 catheter when the stiff back end of a 0.035-in J wire is advanced proximal to the tip. To engage the right coronary ostium with the JL3.5, with the back end of the wire just inside the tip, the catheter is pulled back gently with clockwise torque applied. Once engaged, the wire is removed, and the catheter position usually remains stable.

A few studies have compared the efficiency of the single- versus dual-catheter technique. A Canadian observational study of 1304 patients undergoing TR coronary angiography by 14 different operators compared a dual-catheter technique, primarily Judkins catheters, with a single-catheter strategy. The dual-catheter technique was associated with fewer crossovers, lower radiation exposure, and shorter fluoroscopy time (2.6 vs 2.8 minutes; $P = .03$). Of note, although some Amplatz and multipurpose catheters were used in the single-catheter group, the most frequently used and only "radial-specific" catheter in this study was the

Barbeau catheter, which is not universally used. A randomized study comparing Judkins (JL and JR) with the Tiger catheters demonstrated a significant reduction in procedural and fluoroscopy times by 40% and 33%, respectively, with the latter. RCA and LCA angiograms were completed in 100% and 98% of cases with the Tiger catheter.[7]

GUIDE CATHETER SELECTION FOR TRANSRADIAL CORONARY INTERVENTIONS

The selection of tools for TR catheterization and interventions should take into account some anatomic limitations. The radial artery has a small caliber with a diameter averaging around 2.4 mm (range, 1.8–3 mm).[9] TR PCI cases have been previously described using guides from 4F[10] to 8F catheter.[11] However, most TR interventions can be successfully accomplished with 5F or 6F guiding catheters. All current stent technologies (including covered stents), rotational atherectomy, and/or intravascular ultrasound catheters can be delivered safely and efficiently through 5F to 6F guiding catheters. These guides and equipment still allow for the treatment of simple or even the most complex lesions (ie, bifurcation or chronic total occlusion). Some operators prefer to work through 5F guiding catheters, because the smaller outer diameter is associated with less radial artery injury

and lower incidence of radial artery occlusion.[12] Soft-tip guides can provide greater safety during deep-seating maneuvers.

Guide support is crucial for successful PCI and optimal stent delivery. Inadequate guide backup support accounts for about 17% of the failures for TR-PCI.[4] With the TR approach, either passive or active support of the guiding catheter is important. Active support requires manipulation to obtain a stable, coaxial position, and plays a more important role in TR than in TF intervention. Appropriate choice of guiding catheters, which provide more case-appropriate backup support, is essential to successful TR PCI.

Left Coronary System

Most curves designed for the femoral approach (Judkins, Amplatz, and extra backup catheters) remain well suited for TR PCI. Fig. 6 displays the most frequently used catheters for the LCA. The JL catheters, however, provide less backup support for TR PCI than when used via femoral approach. The angle between the opposite wall of the aorta and the catheter is an important determinant of backup support. The wider the angle between the aortic wall and the catheter, the greater the backup support (Fig. 7). As such, JL catheters are only suited for straightforward interventions for proximal disease where minimal backup support is expected to be required. For ostial left main coronary lesions the Judkins catheters

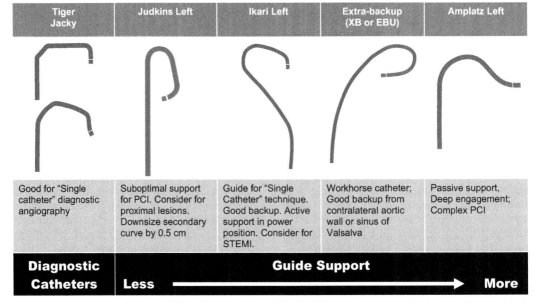

Tiger Jacky	Judkins Left	Ikari Left	Extra-backup (XB or EBU)	Amplatz Left
Good for "Single catheter" diagnostic angiography	Suboptimal support for PCI. Consider for proximal lesions. Downsize secondary curve by 0.5 cm	Guide for "Single Catheter" technique. Good backup. Active support in power position. Consider for STEMI.	Workhorse catheter; Good backup from contralateral aortic wall or sinus of Valsalva	Passive support, Deep engagement; Complex PCI

Diagnostic Catheters	Guide Support	
	Less ⟶	More

Fig. 6. Most common catheters for TR angiography and PCI of the left coronary artery. Optitorque Tiger and Jacky catheter. STEMI, ST elevation myocardial infarction.

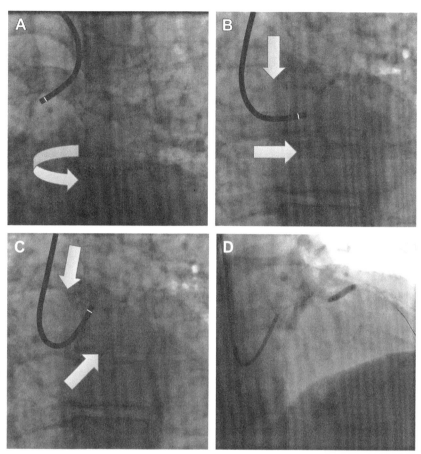

Fig. 7. Left coronary artery cannulation with an extra backup catheter is performed from below the ostium with a counterclockwise movement compared with the more direct and superior cannulation from the femoral route. Engagement is done by advancing the guide to the sinus with the 0.035-in wire (A), then applying torque to point the tip to the left coronary cusp (B). Next, the wire is pulled back and with gentle advancement the catheter engages the left coronary artery (C), after which the operator can proceed with PCI with adequate backup support against the contralateral wall and sinus of Valsalva (D).

remain a good option. For interventions requiring more support, the extra backup catheters (EBU, Voda, or XB) are adequate and remain the most popular. However, a catheter curve that is usually 0.5 cm smaller than what would be used in femoral procedures (3F or 3.5F vs 3.5F or 4F, respectively) may be needed. Engagement into the left main artery is also different from the femoral approach and is cannulated from below the ostium with counterclockwise movement (Fig. 8). These catheters provide passive backup support from the contralateral sinus of Valsalva and offer appropriate deep-seating capability. The Ikari left catheter is an active backup support catheter that allows for a single-catheter strategy to engage both coronaries without sacrificing backup support, which remains comparable with that of extra backup catheters (Fig. 9).

Fine manipulation is usually required to obtain a stable coaxial position in the LCA. This catheter has a similar shape compared with the JL, with three modifications consisting of a shorter secondary curve followed by a straight portion of approximately 20 mm that contacts the contralateral aortic wall providing backup support, a tertiary curve, and a proximal curve to fit the angle between the innominate artery and the aorta. The Ikari left comes in three different curve sizes (3.5, 3.75, and 4), but most cases can be done with the 3.5 curve. In general, it is recommended to use the same curve size as if using a JL catheter.[13]

The Amplatz left catheters (1 or 2) provide great passive backup support and may be the catheters of choice for complex coronary interventions (ie, calcified lesions, chronic total occlusion).

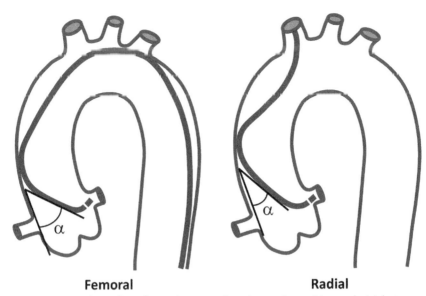

Femoral   **Radial**

Fig. 8. When using a JL catheter from femoral access, there is usually a wider angle (α) between the second segment of the catheter and the contralateral aortic wall. The wider this angle is, the stronger the support, because it allows for more coaxiality and pushability. With TR access this angle is usually narrower with a consequent loss of backup support; therefore, more supportive alternatives for JL catheters, such as extra backup or Amplatz left shapes, are preferred.

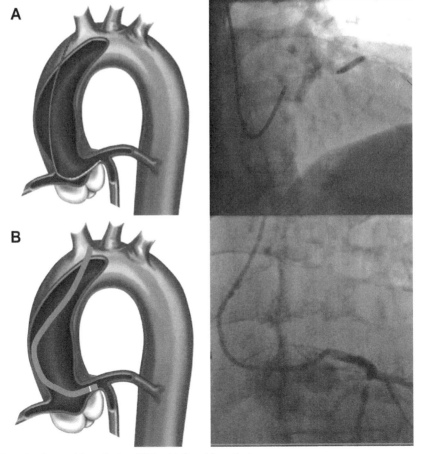

Fig. 9. (A) Extra backup guide catheter. (B) Ikari left guide catheter.

Right Coronary System

The JR guide catheter remains the workhorse catheter used for most TR PCI. It is manipulated in a way similar to that for the femoral approach, with gentle clockwise rotation applied to engage the RCA (Fig. 10). It may be preferred for ostial lesions. However, although the JR catheter shape provides some passive backup, it provides little active backup force because it does not contact the contralateral aortic wall. So although for PCI of "simple" RCA lesions the JR may be adequate, for complex lesions that require additional backup, such as lesions with significant calcification, tortuosity, or chronic occlusions, the JR may be insufficient. A deep coronary intubation can sometimes be helpful for further support and is obtained by careful clockwise rotation and advancement of the guide over an interventional device (wire or balloon) sometimes as deep as the mid segment. But care should be exercised with this aggressive maneuver. Dilated aortic roots and/or RCAs that arise anteriorly also pose a particular problem because the JR catheters often do not have sufficient reach to engage the coronary ostium adequately, coaxial engagement may be limited and PCI may be cumbersome. In this situation, an Amplatz right (1 or 2) or Amplatz left (0.75 or 1) may be a better selection and provide better support. The Amplatz left guide catheter provides further passive support, with more aggressive engagement, which is particularly useful for RCAs with shepherd's crook configuration. Amplatz left catheters may not be the first choice for very proximal or ostial lesions, and carries the risk of catheter-induced traumatic injury to the vessel or aortic wall.

Various catheter shapes have been developed that provide active backup support by contacting with the contralateral aortic wall, and are summarized in Fig. 11. In contrast to the JR catheters, right extra backup guide catheter shapes are also available. The various types of active support curves (Ikari left, EBU-, or XB-RCA type curves) all provide more backup than JR catheters, but have not been compared among each other (Fig. 12). The Ikari left catheter was originally designed for the LCA, but also works well for the RCA. It takes a similar shape to the JR catheter with a 0.035-in guidewire inside. Therefore, the catheter manipulation for engagement is similar to the JR, making it an easy catheter to transition. Unlike the JR, the Ikari left can be pushed further, enhancing the contact with the contralateral aortic wall, and producing greater backup force and a more stable guide position during PCI.[14] Fig. 13 depicts the use of an Ikari left catheter for left and right coronary angiography in a patients with ST elevation myocardial infarction.

Caution should be taken with engagement and manipulation of the Amplatz, Ikari left, and active backup support catheters. The Ikari left in the RCA may engage deeply at the power position. Coaxial alignment should be maintained to avoid the risk of traumatic, iatrogenic dissections, although the incidence remains low. Care should also be taken because respiratory variation could lead to back-and-forth catheter motion and displacement of coaxial positioning at the ostium of the RCA.

There are also various additional radial-specific guide catheters including the Kimny, Barbeau, and Fadajet catheters that are effective for RCA PCI. These unique shapes have been designed and developed by radial pioneers, remain less frequently used, and require some additional degree of expertise with manipulation

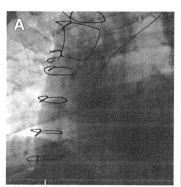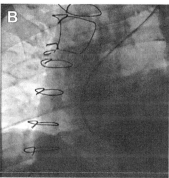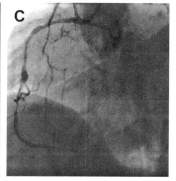

Fig. 10. Right coronary artery cannulation with a Judkins right catheter is performed by advancing the catheter to the aortic valve cusps (A). With the catheter tip horizontal above the aortic valve plane the catheter is continued in a clockwise rotation (B) until engaged into the RCA (C).

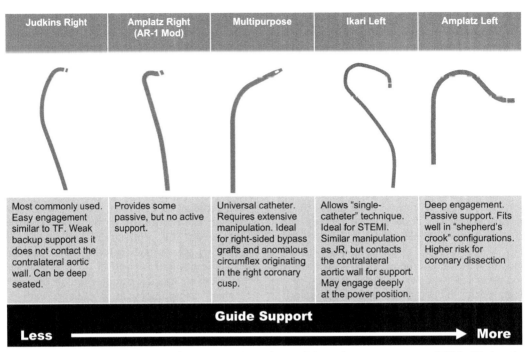

Judkins Right	Amplatz Right (AR-1 Mod)	Multipurpose	Ikari Left	Amplatz Left
Most commonly used. Easy engagement similar to TF. Weak backup support as it does not contact the contralateral aortic wall. Can be deep seated.	Provides some passive, but no active support.	Universal catheter. Requires extensive manipulation. Ideal for right-sided bypass grafts and anomalous circumflex originating in the right coronary cusp.	Allows "single-catheter" technique. Ideal for STEMI. Similar manipulation as JR, but contacts the contralateral aortic wall for support. May engage deeply at the power position.	Deep engagement. Passive support. Fits well in "shepherd's crook" configurations. Higher risk for coronary dissection

Guide Support

Less ➝ **More**

Fig. 11. Most common TR catheters for angiography and PCI of the right coronary artery. STEMI, ST elevation myocardial infarction.

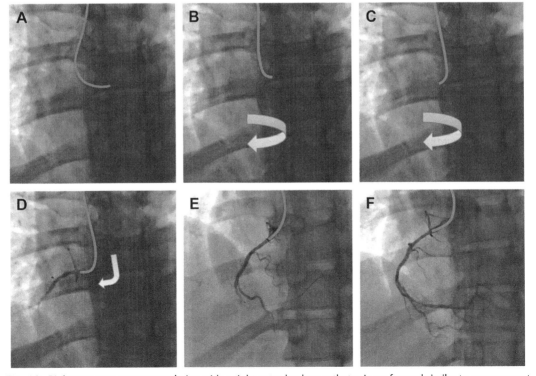

Fig. 12. Right coronary artery cannulation with a right extra backup catheter is performed similar to engagement with a JR catheter. With the catheter tip horizontal above the aortic valve plane (A), the catheter is rotated clockwise (B, C) until engaged into the RCA (D). Coaxial alignment and contralateral backup support (E) allow for PCI and wire crossing of a CTO and provide enough support to successfully deliver equipment (F) and successfully complete PCI.

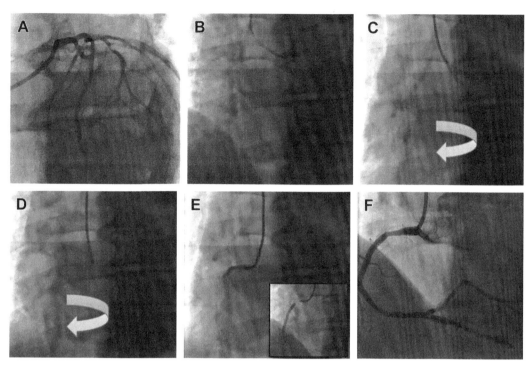

Fig. 13. During TR primary PCI both coronary vessels can be easily imaged with a single-catheter strategy using the Ikari left catheter. After LCA angiography using an Ikari left guide (*A*) proceeded to engage the RCA by clockwise rotation (*B–D*). Angiography demonstrated a mid RCA occlusion (*E*). After thrombectomy and stenting (*inset*, *E*), the final result showed final TIMI 3 flow in the RCA (*F*).

for use. The Kimny catheter has a 45-degree primary curve and a 90-degree secondary curve, which provides contralateral backup support and can be used to cannulate both coronary arteries.[15] The RCA is cannulated from a horizontal or superior position, and may be useful in particular for Shepherd's hook RCA origin. The Barbeau catheter is essentially a modified multipurpose catheter with an additional 135-degree curve at the tip. Cannulation of the RCA with this catheter is performed by manipulating from above the ostium with a clockwise "corkscrew" maneuver.

Saphenous Vein Bypass Grafts
The performance of an aortic root angiogram may be advisable before engagement of saphenous vein grafts to better understand the type of catheter shapes that are needed. There are minor differences in saphenous vein graft engagement depending on right or left TR access, right TR access being somewhat more technically challenging. For left-sided vein grafts, although a JR4 may still function well, left coronary bypass or Amplatz type guiding catheters are better suited with better reach to the anterior left and anterior

aortic wall. For right-sided vein grafts, a JR4 guiding catheter may be adequate. In the setting of a downward oriented, right-sided saphenous vein graft, a multipurpose guiding catheter may prove better. In general, left TR access provides better backup support for right-sided grafts compared with right TR access.[16]

Internal Mammary Artery Grafts
Although the right radial approach is used in at least 90% of all TR cases performed, the left radial approach is more suitable in patients with prior coronary artery bypass graft involving the left internal mammary artery (LIMA).[17] Ipsilateral access to internal mammary artery grafts is easiest and cannulation of the LIMA graft is best approached via the left TR approach. Either a modified or nonmodified mammary guide catheter may be used. In the rare case when left TR is not possible, such as where the left radial artery has been used for a bypass conduit, or in patients of double mammary grafts, engagement of the left internal mammary is still possible from the right radial approach.[16,18] Accessing the contralateral internal mammary artery is technically challenging. The steps to

engage the LIMA from right TR access include the following (Fig. 14):

- A catheter (JR4 usually works best) is maneuvered over the wire to the aortic arch.
- The catheter tip is then torqued gently to engage upward into the left subclavian artery.
- A soft hydrophilic wire can then be advanced far distally into axillary/brachial artery.
- The wire can be fixed by bending the elbow or by inflating a blood pressure cuff on the left arm.
- The catheter initially used to advance the wire into the left subclavian artery is exchanged for a soft 4F internal mammary (IM) catheter that tracks over the trapped wire without prolapsing into the descending aorta.
- Once the catheter reaches the left subclavian artery distal to the origin of the LIMA, the wire is removed and the catheter is pulled gently and torqued counterclockwise searching for the LIMA ostium. The best view to perform this maneuver is 10-degree right anterior oblique with some degree of cranial angulation.

Right internal mammary artery (RIMA) bypass grafts can be straightforward to access via right TR access. However, the origin of the RIMA ostium often sits perpendicular to the catheter plane, making it harder to engage. A VB-1 internal mammary artery catheter has a more acutely angulated tip, similar to a fish hook, and may be helpful in this case. Another technique, which has been described to facilitate engagement of the RIMA, involves reshaping the catheter tip by bending and collapsing it in the subclavian or innominate artery. Alternatively, any standard 0.014-in coronary guidewire can be used to wire the RIMA, and anchor and engage the guide by tracking the catheter over it.

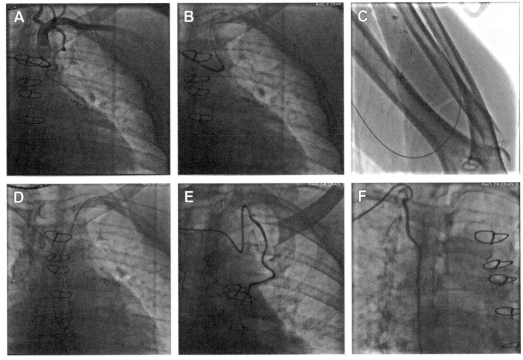

Fig. 14. To engage LIMA from the contralateral radial approach, a 5F or 6F catheter is pointed toward the left subclavian artery (A), then a soft, angled-tip hydrophilic wire is advanced into the left subclavian artery (B) as far as possible into the left upper extremity. The wire can be stabilized by inflating a blood pressure cuff or asking the patient to flex the elbow (C). Then the initial 5F to 6F catheter is exchanged for a soft 4F IM catheter, which is slowly advanced into the subclavian artery sometimes finding support in the sinuses of Valsalva (D). Once the catheter tip reaches past the origin of the LIMA, the wire can be removed. Gentle torqueing while carefully pulling the catheter allows selective LIMA cannulation (E). The RIMA can be selectively engaged with a modified IM VB-1 catheter (F).

Anomalous Coronary Arteries and Transradial Interventions

Certain coronary anomalies or variants, albeit infrequent, are worth mentioning. An anterior take-off of the RCA may require additional catheter length and support, which is often best provided using an Amplatz left catheter. Similarly, the Amplatz left catheters (1 or 2) work similarly well for anomalous RCA arising from the left cusp. However, when engagement is difficult, a technique previously described for the TF approach can also be used with TR access using a catheter with larger secondary curve than the one used to cannulate the LCA ostium, such as a JL4 or JL5 or even a Tiger catheter. The catheter is pushed deep into the left coronary sinus, causing it to make an anterior and upward "U-turn." The loop created prevents the catheter from engaging the LCA, allowing for selective cannulation of an anomalous RCA.[19] JR5 and multipurpose catheters are helpful to engage anomalous circumflex arteries originating from the right coronary sinus.

OPTIMIZING GUIDE CATHETER SUPPORT DURING TRANSRADIAL PERCUTANEOUS CORONARY INTERVENTIONS

Even with coaxial engagement, additional support is occasionally needed during TR PCI because of different anatomic configurations of the aortic arch. Various maneuvers to obtain additional support have been described including deep intubation, use of "active backup catheters," "mother-child" catheter-in-catheter technique, anchoring balloons, or buddy wire techniques.

Deep intubation of the coronary artery can reliably be obtained with soft-tip and smaller-diameter guide catheters. However, this carries a risk of traumatic injury to the proximal vessel, particularly if there is significant disease. In some situations, a larger guide catheter may provide more stability and "passive backup." A buddy wire, a stiffer extrasupport wire, or placing a second stiff wire in the left anterior descending while intervening in the left circumflex (or vice versa) may also be useful for further support.[20] An anchoring balloon can be placed in a proximal small side branch and inflated at low pressure during advancement of interventional devices. A "mother-child" hybrid system has also been proposed as a way to enhance the backup support of 6F catheters and also allow for the use of smaller guide catheters to perform deep intubation maneuvers to treat lesions with extreme proximal tortuosity or heavy calcification. A "five-in-six" system in which a 5F, 120-cm long guide catheter is inserted into a 6F, 100-cm long guide catheter has been described.[21] Subsequently, a "four-in-six" system was attempted, which demonstrated superior trackability and better backup support with high rates of technical success.[22] An analogous option is the use of extension catheters, such as the GuideLiner (Vascular Solutions, Inc, Minneapolis, MN) or Guidezilla (Boston Scientific, Marlborough, MA) (Fig. 15).[23,24] These devices are a "rapid-exchange" version of the mother-child system and consist of a 20-cm soft-tipped catheter connected with a metal collar to a 115-cm stainless steel shaft for advancement and positioning. These extensions allow for safer, deep intubation of the target vessel, which provides additional support during complex PCI when there is difficulty in advancing equipment, such as balloon and/or stents across the target lesion. Additionally, for PCI of chronic total occlusion it can help reestablish a reentry plane in the case of retrograde crossing or reverse controlled antegrade and retrograde subintimal tracking.

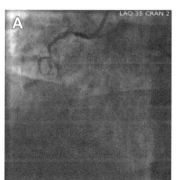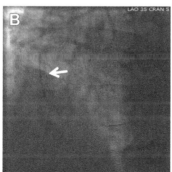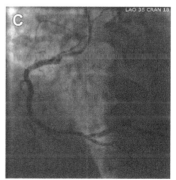

Fig. 15. In this example of a CTO intervention (*A–C*), additional support in a tortuous and calcified vessel is needed to advance further balloons and/or stents. A specialty catheter extension device, such as the Guideliner (*arrow* in *B*), is useful in this scenario in addition to a strong passive backup catheter, such as an Amplatz left.

SUMMARY

TR PCI confers various well-documented benefits over femoral coronary angiography and PCI. Most coronary procedures can be performed safely and effectively using the TR approach. Certain anatomic variants pose additional challenges, but these can usually be identified and overcome. Guiding catheters of 6F catheter are sufficient for most interventions, and the shape should be selected based on the anticipated required guide support. Active backup support catheters should be considered for more complex anatomy. Larger catheters can be used in select complex PCI cases using a sheathless approach. Despite various dedicated radial shapes, the standard-shaped guide catheters still remain most common and sufficient for most cases. Universal radial catheters and single-catheter approaches may offer some further potential benefits compared with standard shapes. A single-catheter approach has the potential to further decrease the duration of procedures, radiation exposure, and contrast volume, and may be ideally suited for ST elevation myocardial infarction interventions. No one guide catheter has shown to be superior to others. Rather, guide catheter selection is operator dependent minding the clinical scenario and anatomic considerations at hand. Guide catheter selection and manipulation remains a key component of successful TR catheterization and coronary intervention.

REFERENCES

1. Rao SV, Cohen MG, Kandzari DE, et al. The transradial approach to percutaneous coronary intervention: historical perspective, current concepts, and future directions. J Am Coll Cardiol 2010;55:2187–95.
2. Bertrand OF, Belisle P, Joyal D, et al. Comparison of transradial and femoral approaches for percutaneous coronary interventions: a systematic review and hierarchical Bayesian meta-analysis. Am Heart J 2012;163:632–48.
3. Jolly SS, Amlani S, Hamon M, et al. Radial versus femoral access for coronary angiography or intervention and the impact on major bleeding and ischemic events: a systematic review and meta-analysis of randomized trials. Am Heart J 2009; 157:132–40.
4. Dehghani P, Mohammad A, Bajaj R, et al. Mechanism and predictors of failed transradial approach for percutaneous coronary interventions. JACC Cardiovasc Interv 2009;2:1057–64.
5. Yiu KH, Chan WS, Jim MH, et al. Arteria lusoria diagnosed by transradial coronary catheterization. JACC Cardiovasc Interv 2010;3:880–1.

6. Ruiz-Salmeron RJ, Mora R, Velez-Gimon M, et al. Radial artery spasm in transradial cardiac catheterization. Assessment of factors related to its occurrence, and of its consequences during follow-up. Rev Esp Cardiol 2005;58:504–11 [in Spanish]
7. Kim SM, Kim DK, Kim DI, et al. Novel diagnostic catheter specifically designed for both coronary arteries via the right transradial approach. A prospective, randomized trial of Tiger II vs Judkins catheters. Int J Cardiovasc Imaging 2006;22:295–303.
8. Freestone B, Nolan J. Transradial cardiac procedures: the state of the art. Heart 2010;96:883–91.
9. Saito S, Ikei H, Hosokawa G, et al. Influence of the ratio between radial artery inner diameter and sheath outer diameter on radial artery flow after transradial coronary intervention. Catheter Cardiovasc Interv 1999;46:173–8.
10. Takeshita S, Shiono T, Takagi A, et al. Percutaneous coronary intervention using a novel 4-French coronary accessor. Catheter Cardiovasc Interv 2008;72: 222–7.
11. Metz D, Meyer P, Touati C, et al. Comparison of 6F with 7F and 8F guiding catheters for elective coronary angioplasty: results of a prospective, multicenter, randomized trial. Am Heart J 1997;134: 131–7.
12. Dahm JB, Vogelgesang D, Hummel A, et al. A randomized trial of 5 vs 6 French transradial percutaneous coronary interventions. Catheter Cardiovasc Interv 2002;57:172–6.
13. Ikari Y, Nagaoka M, Kim JY, et al. The physics of guiding catheters for the left coronary artery in transfemoral and transradial interventions. J Invasive Cardiol 2005;17:636–41.
14. Ikari Y, Masuda N, Matsukage T, et al. Backup force of guiding catheters for the right coronary artery in transfemoral and transradial interventions. J Invasive Cardiol 2009;21:570–4.
15. Shibata Y, Doi O, Goto T, et al. New guiding catheter for transrad PTCA. Cathet Cardiovasc Diagn 1998;43:344–51.
16. Burzotta F, Trani C, Hamon M, et al. Transradial approach for coronary angiography and interventions in patients with coronary bypass grafts: tips and tricks. Catheter Cardiovasc Interv 2008;72: 263–72.
17. Bertrand OF, Rao SV, Pancholy S, et al. Transradial approach for coronary angiography and interventions: results of the first international transradial practice survey. JACC Cardiovasc Interv 2010;3: 1022–31.
18. Patel T, Shah S, Patel T. Cannulating LIMA graft using right transradial approach: two simple and innovative techniques. Catheter Cardiovasc Interv 2012;80:316–20.
19. Cohen MG, Tolleson TR, Peter RH, et al. Successful percutaneous coronary intervention with stent

implantation in anomalous right coronary arteries arising from the left sinus of valsalva: a report of two cases. Catheter Cardiovasc Interv 2002;55:105–8.

20. Dana A, Barbeau GR. The use of multiple "buddies" during transradial angioplasty in a complex calcified coronary tree. Catheter Cardiovasc Interv 2006;67:396–9.

21. Takahashi S, Saito S, Tanaka S, et al. New method to increase a backup support of a 6 French guiding coronary catheter. Catheter Cardiovasc Interv 2004; 63:452–6.

22. Takeshita S, Shishido K, Sugitatsu K, et al. In vitro and human studies of a 4F double-coaxial

technique ("mother-child" configuration) to facilitate stent implantation in resistant coronary vessels. Circ Cardiovasc Interv 2011;4:155–61.

23. Farooq V, Mamas MA, Fath-Ordoubadi F, et al. The use of a guide catheter extension system as an aid during transradial percutaneous coronary intervention of coronary artery bypass grafts. Catheter Cardiovasc Interv 2011;78:847–63.

24. Moynagh A, Garot P, Lefevre T, et al. Angiographic success and successful stent delivery for complex lesions using the GuideLiner five-in-six system- a case report. Am Heart Hosp J 2011;9: E44–7.

Slender Approach and Sheathless Techniques

Saurabh Sanon, MD, Rajiv Gulati, MD, PhD*

KEYWORDS

• Radial artery • Sheathless • Slender • Transradial intervention • Percutaneous coronary intervention

KEY POINTS

• Most radial arteries cannot accommodate 7-French (F) and 8F introducer sheaths for large-bore percutaneous coronary intervention (PCI) without overstretch.
• In addition to being uncomfortable, radial artery overstretch is associated with spasm and higher rates of procedure-related radial artery occlusion.
• Methods for the transradial interventionist to overcome the limitation of radial artery–sheath size mismatch include both sheath-based and sheathless approaches.
• Slender techniques can be used to minimize radial stretch for standard coronary procedures.

INTRODUCTION

Despite the clinical benefits of transradial compared with transfemoral intervention,[1–3] the narrow caliber of the radial artery compared with the femoral artery has historically been considered a limitation for the performance of complex PCI. Yoo and colleagues[4] reported the inner diameter of the radial artery to be smaller than the outer diameter of a 7F introducer sheath in 75% of patients. Moreover, Saito and colleagues[5] suggested that the radial artery was of smaller diameter than standard 6F introducer sheaths in 27.4% of women and 14.3% of men. Thus, most radial arteries cannot accommodate 7F and 8F introducer sheaths for large-bore PCI without overstretch. In addition to being uncomfortable, radial artery overstretch is associated with spasm and higher rates of procedure-related radial artery occlusion.[5–10]

This article discusses practical methods for the transradial interventionist to overcome the limitation of radial artery–sheath size mismatch. These strategies include both sheath-based and sheathless approaches. An adaptation of sheathless techniques also allows for the performance of minimally invasive (slender) PCI, where the radial artery is only exposed to stretch from 5F and 6F guiding catheters equating to the outer diameters of 3F and 4F introducer sheaths.

SHEATH-BASED APPROACHES

The In-Out Method

The in-out method uses a standard large-bore introducer sheath, typically 7F (Fig. 1). The method minimizes overstretch by, first, affecting only the most distal 1 to 2 cm of the accessed radial artery and, second, being in place for only enough time to introduce the guiding catheter, typically a few seconds:

1. The wrist is prepped 360° and a compression band is put in place, left unstrapped, and ready for later use.
2. A 7F sheath is cut to 2 cm in length (see Fig. 1A).
3. The shortened sheath is inserted with its dilator over a 0.035-in wire in the radial artery (see Fig. 1B).
4. The sheath dilator is removed and a 7F guiding catheter is advanced to the coronary artery.
5. The compression band is strapped in place and the shortened sheath removed. To

The authors have nothing to disclose.
Division of Cardiovascular Diseases, Mayo Clinic, 200 First Street Southwest, Rochester, MN 55905, USA
* Corresponding author.
E-mail address: gulati.rajiv@mayo.edu

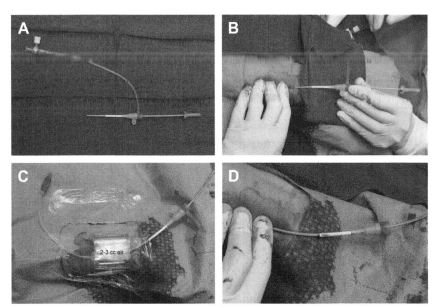

Fig. 1. In-out method. (A) A standard 7F introducer sheath is cut short to approximately 2 cm. (B) The dilator-sheath setup is advanced into the radial artery over a 0.035-in wire in a standard manner. The sheath dilator is removed and a guiding catheter advanced. Site ooze can be controlled with a (C) compression band or (D) gentle manual pressure.

prevent ooze from the radial arteriotomy site at this stage, the compression band can be inflated with 2 to 3 mL of air (see Fig. 1C) and the band can be deflated after 1 to 2 minutes. Alternatively 1 to 2 minutes of gentle manual pressure can be applied instead of the compression band (see Fig. 1D).

Thin-Walled Sheaths

Recently developed thin-walled sheaths (Glide-sheath Slender, Terumo, Somerset, New Jersey) are an excellent way of pursuing large-bore or standard-bore transradial intervention (TRI) without new techniques and without changes to standard workflow. Standard sheaths have in effect been cored out such that their walls are now thinner.

The 6F-in-5F radial sheath thus has an internal working lumen compatible with a 6F guide but an outside diameter equivalent to a 5F sheath (Fig. 2). Similarly, the 7F-in-6F sheath can accommodate a 7F guide while itself having the outer diameter of a standard-walled 6F sheath. In contrast to femoral sheaths that require a thicker wall to prevent kinking when bent while traversing tissue, radial sheaths usually require traversing a smaller tissue thickness and enter the artery at a relatively acute angle, thereby allowing the use of thinner walls without compromising sheath performance. Aminian and

colleagues[11] studied the use of this sheath in 114 patients undergoing transradial angiography and reported a success rate of 99.1% with a 4.4% rate of radial artery spasm and 0.88% rate of radial artery occlusion at 1 month. The availability of such dedicated radial sheaths allows performance of slender PCI without the need to use dedicated sheathless guides or homemade sheathless guide systems.

SHEATHLESS SYSTEMS

An important concern when introducing a sheathless guide is the potential for damage to the arterial entry site due to lack of a smooth taper at the guide tip (Fig. 3A). Commercial systems and homemade strategies can be used to address this concern. Another theoretic limitation is trauma to the unprotected radial artery if excessive torquing of the guiding catheter is required. This could result in spasm or increase the risk of trauma-induced radial occlusion.

Commercial Sheathless Guide System

Commercial sheathless guide system catheters are available in 6.5F and 7.5F sizes, with outer diameters of 2.16 mm and 2.49 mm approximating those of 5F and 6F introducer sheaths (see Fig. 3, Eaucath, Asahi Intecc, Aichi, Japan). Each guide, available in a variety of tip shapes, is packaged with a long dilator. The dilators have been fashioned to taper tightly over a 0.035-in

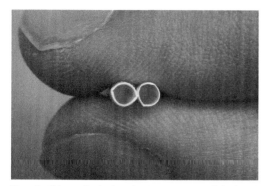

Fig. 2. Thin-walled sheath. A 6-in, 5F Glidesheath Slender (*right*) has a thinner wall compared with a standard sheath (*left*). Both sheaths have the same outer diameter, but the Glidesheath Slender has a larger inner diameter and is thus able to accommodate a larger caliber guide.

wire at the distal end as well as to fit snugly in the guiding catheter at its tip (see Fig. 3B). The guide-dilator setup is then advanced over an exchange length 0.035-in wire in the radial artery (see Fig. 3C). Once in the ascending aorta, the dilator can be removed over the wire (see Fig. 3D). The smooth transitions (wire-dilator and dilator-guide, see Fig. 3A) result in minimal

trauma to the radial arteriotomy site on advancement. The guiding catheters have a hydrophilic coating along the entire length for easy advancement. The coating may raise propensity for guiding catheter slippage, either backwards (thereby disengaging from the coronary) or forwards (risk of coronary trauma). A transparent adhesive dressing applied over the radial entry site after guide engagement may help mitigate this risk. Cost remains another consideration for widespread uptake.[12,13]

Homemade Sheathless Systems

The authors' group and other investigators have used homemade sheathless systems to be used with standard guiding catheters. The following are methods used to create a pseudotaper at the guide tip for easy guide insertion into the radial artery (Fig. 4). Due to the variety of sizes available for each of the pseudotapers, the methods can be adopted for large-bore (7F and 8F) guides and to minimize radial stretch with standard guides (slender approach, 5F and 6F guides).

- Use a partially inflated coronary balloon at the guide tip and insert this over a stiff 0.014-in exchange length coronary guide wire (see Fig. 4A).

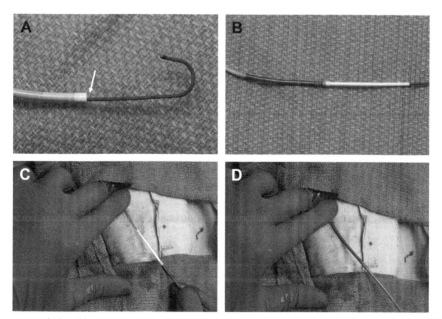

Fig. 3. Commercial sheathless system. (*A*) Razor edge (*arrow*) of standard guiding catheter over 0.035-in wire would result in significant trauma to the radial artery entry site if entry attempted. (*B*) Long tapered dilator allows for tight fit over a 0.035-in wire and snug hold at guide tip, thereby providing a smooth transition for guide insertion. (*C*) Dilator and guide are advanced over a 0.035-in wire. (*D*) Dilator can be removed from ascending aorta, leaving sheathless guide in place.

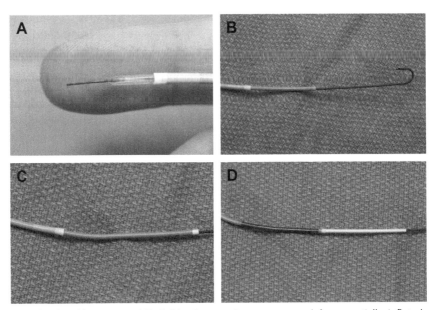

Fig. 4. Homemade sheathless setup. (A) Guide tip pseudotapers created from partially inflated angioplasty balloon over a 0.014-in coronary guide wire; (B) GuideLiner extension catheter over a 0.035-in guide wire; (C) 5F, 125-cm diagnostic multipurpose catheter inserted through a 6F guide over a 0.035-in guide wire; and (D) 4F, 110-cm sheath dilator within a 5F guiding catheter over a 0.035-in guide wire.

- A guide extension (GuideLiner, Vascular Solutions, Minneapolis, MN) through a standard and over a 0.035-in guide wire (see Fig. 4B).
- A 125-cm Multipurpose diagnostic catheter inserted within a guiding catheter 1F size larger. Example shown is a 5F diagnostic within a 6F guide catheter (see Fig. 4C).
- A 5F, 125-cm Shuttle Select diagnostic catheter (Cordis, Fremont, CA) through a 6F guiding catheter inserted over a 0.035-in guide wire. Similarly, a 6.5F Shuttle Select catheter (Cordis) fits snugly within an 8F guide.
- A 110-cm 4F sheath dilator (Check-Flo, Cook Medical, Bloomington, IN) within a 5F guiding catheter with (see Fig. 4D).
- A Corsair microcatheter (Asahi, Tokyo, Japan), which has a smooth tapered tip, through a 5F guiding catheter over a 0.014-in guide wire.

After the authors' feasibility studies, Kwan and colleagues[14] extended evaluation of these strategies and reported a 100% success rate using balloon-assisted sheathless TRI using a sheathless 5F guiding catheter (n = 27). The same group also studied the feasibility and safety of large-bore sheathless guiding catheter use for TRI in 116 patients and reported a success rate of 95%, with radial artery occlusion rates of 5% and 2.5%, at 7 days and 30 days, respectively. Approximately 50% of these were complex interventions, including chronic total occlusions (CTOs), bifurcation stenting, and calcified lesions.[15]

SLENDER TRANSRADIAL TECHNIQUES

Slender techniques focus on maximal miniaturization of TRI and utilize specially designed thin-walled sheaths as well as commercial or homemade small-bore sheathless guide systems. The application, benefits, and limitations of these techniques are discussed.

Slender Transradial Intervention (Virtual 3 French)

The slender movement, beginning in Japan, has focused on performing transradial angiography and TRI with the minimum possible internal stretch pressure to the radial artery wall. Current techniques involve using a sheathless 5F guiding catheter, which has an outside diameter equivalent to a 3F sheath but an internal working lumen of a 5F system (often called the virtual 3F method).[16,17] Intravascular ultrasound using an Eagle Eye catheter (Volcano Corporation, San Diego, California) and a 0.014-in guide wire and fractional flow reserve are both possible as well as PCI with up to a 4-mm diameter stent via such a virtual 3F system. Tonomura and colleagues[17] evaluated the feasibility of this technique in 132 patients undergoing TRI and reported a 95% success rate and a 4.5%

conversion rate (6 of 132 patients) to a conventional 5F or 6F system. Approximately one-third of the lesions intervened on were complex (type B2 or C) in this study. To enhance guide support and facilitate device delivery with this system, other investigators have reported using a 4-in-3 slender mother and child technique wherein a 4F straight guiding catheter is introduced in a virtual 3F system to successfully complete TRI.[18] Using this small-caliber system, the incidence of skin and endovascular trauma is minimized (comparable to that caused by a 3F sheath), and patient comfort is enhanced while maintaining the ability to perform simple and relatively complex coronary interventions.

Limitations of virtual 3F systems include the inability to deliver stents greater than 4 mm in diameter or cutting balloons greater than 3 mm in size and the inability to perform bifurcation stenting or delivering simultaneous devices. Manual aspiration thrombectomy requires a 6F compatible system and also cannot be performed; however, deep vessel intubation with 5F guides can be performed for directly manual aspiration. Kissing balloon dilation is not possible using a standard 0.014-in guide wire; however, it becomes feasible using a 0.010-in guide wire compatible system available in some countries. Matsukage and colleagues[19] demonstrated the safety and feasibility of the 0.010-in compatible system and reported a stent delivery success rate of 93.9% using this setup. CTO revascularization generally requires larger guides and more backup support; however, short CTOs with favorable characteristics might be amenable to revascularization using slender techniques. Moreover, the slender technique can be used in retrograde CTO revascularization because microcatheters, such as the Corsair catheter, can be inserted through a 5F system. Mizuno and colleagues[20] treated 36 coronary lesions, including 7 CTOs, using a virtual 3F system and reported a success rate of 92%, with no access site complications or radial artery occlusion. Other limitations of virtual 3F TRI include the need for cumbersome guide catheter exchange over an exchange length guide wire, in the event that the catheter fails to engage the vessel or provide adequate support; the additional care that is warranted to prevent air entrapment during wire exchanges; and meticulous catheter flushing to prevent thrombus formation within the small-caliber system.

SUMMARY

Sheath-based and sheathless approaches can be used to minimize stretch to the radial artery during angiography intervention. These approaches allow for complex TRI using large-bore guides without resulting in prolonged radial overstretch. Similarly, slender techniques can be used to minimize radial stretch for standard coronary procedures.

REFERENCES

1. Kiemeneij F, Laarman GJ, Odekerken D, et al. A randomized comparison of percutaneous transluminal coronary angioplasty by the radial, brachial and femoral approaches: the access study. J Am Coll Cardiol 1997;29:1269–75.

2. Romagnoli E, Biondi-Zoccai G, Sciahbasi A, et al. Radial versus femoral randomized investigation in ST-segment elevation acute coronary syndrome: the RIFLE-STEACS (Radial Versus Femoral Randomized Investigation in ST-Elevation Acute Coronary Syndrome) study. J Am Coll Cardiol 2012;60:2481–9.

3. Agostoni P, Biondi-Zoccai GG, de Benedictis ML, et al. Radial versus femoral approach for percutaneous coronary diagnostic and interventional procedures; Systematic overview and meta-analysis of randomized trials. J Am Coll Cardiol 2004;44:349–56.

4. Yoo BS, Yoon J, Ko JY, et al. Anatomical consideration of the radial artery for transradial coronary procedures: arterial diameter, branching anomaly and vessel tortuosity. Int J Cardiol 2005;101:421–7.

5. Saito S, Ikei H, Hosokawa G, et al. Influence of the ratio between radial artery inner diameter and sheath outer diameter on radial artery flow after transradial coronary intervention. Catheter Cardiovasc Interv 1999;46:173–8.

6. Dahm JB, Vogelgesang D, Hummel A, et al. A randomized trial of 5 vs. 6 French transradial percutaneous coronary interventions. Catheter Cardiovasc Interv 2002;57:172–6.

7. Jia DA, Zhou YJ, Shi DM, et al. Incidence and predictors of radial artery spasm during transradial coronary angiography and intervention. Chin Med J 2010;123:843–7.

8. Sakai H, Ikeda S, Harada T, et al. Limitations of successive transradial approach in the same arm: the Japanese experience. Catheter Cardiovasc Interv 2001;54:204–8.

9. From AM, Bell MR, Rihal CS, et al. Minimally invasive transradial intervention using sheathless standard guiding catheters. Catheter Cardiovasc Interv 2011;78:866–71.

10. From AM, Gulati R, Prasad A, et al. Sheathless transradial intervention using standard guide catheters. Catheter Cardiovasc Interv 2010;76:911–6.

11. Aminian A, Dolatabadi D, Lefebvre P, et al. Initial experience with the glidesheath slender for

transradial coronary angiography and intervention: a feasibility study with prospective radial ultrasound follow-up. Catheter Cardiovasc Interv 2014; 84:438–42.

12. Cogliano MA, Tolerico PH. Nonhealing wound resulting from a foreign body to a radial arterial sheath and sterile inflammation associated with transradial catheterization and hydrophilic sheaths. Catheter Cardiovasc Interv 2004;63: 104–5.

13. Kozak M, Adams DR, Ioffreda MD, et al. Sterile inflammation associated with transradial catheterization and hydrophilic sheaths. Catheter Cardiovasc Interv 2003;59:207–13.

14. Kwan TW, Ratcliffe JA, Huang Y, et al. Balloon-assisted sheathless transradial intervention (BASTI) using 5 Fr guiding catheters. J Invasive Cardiol 2012;24:231–3.

15. Kwan TW, Cherukuri S, Huang Y, et al. Feasibility and safety of 7F sheathless guiding catheter during transradial coronary intervention. Catheter Cardiovasc Interv 2012;80:274–80.

16. Matsukage T, Yoshimachi F, Masutani M, et al. Virtual 3 Fr PCI system for complex percutaneous coronary intervention. EuroIntervention 2009;5:515–7.

17. Tonomura D, Shimada Y, Yano K, et al. Feasibility and safety of a virtual 3-Fr sheathless-guiding system for percutaneous coronary intervention. Catheter Cardiovasc Interv 2014;84:426–35.

18. Honda T, Fujimoto K, Miyao Y. Successful percutaneous coronary intervention using a 4-in-3 "Slender Mother and Child" PCI technique. Postepy Kardiol Interwencyjnej 2013;9:286–90.

19. Matsukage T, Yoshimachi F, Masutani M, et al. A new 0.010-inch guidewire and compatible balloon catheter system: the IKATEN registry. Catheter Cardiovasc Interv 2009;73:605–10.

20. Mizuno S, Takeshita S, Taketani Y, et al. Percutaneous coronary intervention using a virtual 3-Fr guiding catheter. Catheter Cardiovasc Interv 2010;75:983–8.

Transradial Primary Percutaneous Coronary Intervention

Sasko Kedev, MD, PhD, FESC, FACC

KEYWORDS

- Transradial approach • ST segment elevation myocardial infarction • Acute coronary syndrome
- Percutaneous coronary intervention • Transfemoral approach • Bleeding complications

KEY POINTS

- Bleeding complications remain an important cause of morbidity and mortality in patients with acute ST segment elevation myocardial infarction (STEMI) undergoing primary percutaneous coronary intervention (PPCI).
- Access-site bleeding is greatest among the STEMI population.
- Transradial access PPCI is associated with significant reduction in bleeding and vascular complications and with lower mortality compared with the transfemoral approach (TFA).
- Specific radial skills providing procedural times and success rates comparable with those of the TFA are strongly recommended before using this technique in the STEMI PPCI setting.
- A stepwise approach to learning is proposed and high-risk STEMI percutaneous coronary intervention is recommended as the last step.
- A team approach to patient management is crucial in the catheterization laboratory.

 Videos of right forearm angiogram demonstrating significant radial artery tortuosity and tortuosity negotiated with 0.014-inch guidewire accompany this article at http://www.interventional.theclinics.com/

INTRODUCTION

Primary percutaneous coronary intervention (PPCI) improves clinical outcomes in patients with ST segment elevation myocardial infarction (STEMI) and in high-risk patients with non–ST segment elevation acute coronary syndrome (NSTEACS).[1,2] The transfemoral approach (TFA) is still the most widely used percutaneous access site in most cardiac catheterization laboratories worldwide. However, being a deep and terminal vessel the femoral artery may expose the patient to frequent bleeding and vascular complications,[3,4] especially in the setting of STEMI, in which potent antithrombotic drugs are frequently used.[5,6] Since its initial description as a safe and feasible access route for cardiac catheterization,[7,8] transradial access (TRA) has increasingly been used for percutaneous coronary intervention (PCI). The main advantage compared with TFA is a reduced risk of access-site bleeding and major vascular complications, particularly in the presence of multiple and more powerful antiplatelet and antithrombotic agents.[9] This risk is mainly related to the more favorable anatomy of the radial artery, which runs superficially, separated from major neurovascular structures, thus allowing shorter times to hemostasis and ambulation compared with TFA.[10]

Disclosure: The author has nothing to disclose.
Medical Faculty, University Clinic of Cardiology, University of St. Cyril & Methodius, Vodnjanska 17, Skopje 1000, Macedonia
E-mail address: skedev@gmail.com

More recently, the radial approach has been associated with mortality benefits for patients with STEMI and with reduction in mortality, myocardial infarction (MI), and stroke for patients undergoing the procedure at high-volume radial centers[11–13]

Reported access failure for radial procedures in PPCI is low, with an access crossover rate between 3.8%[14] and 9.6%[13] with negligible time delay with expert operators. There are several reasons leading to failure: inability to cannulate, severe radial artery spasm (RAS), and anatomic variations. In some of these difficult transradial cases, ulnar artery cannulation has been proposed as a reasonable and useful alternative to TRA if performed by an experienced radial operator, before crossover to TFA.[15,16]

BLEEDING COMPLICATIONS IN ACUTE CORONARY SYNDROME

Periprocedural PPCI bleeding complications have consistently been associated with worse outcomes and increased short-term and long-term mortality.[6,17] Access site–related bleeding, accounting for as many as 30% to 50% of all causes of bleeding in patients with acute coronary syndrome (ACS), are the major contributor for bleeding events.[9,18–20]

Because of the firm link between bleeding, ischemic events, and mortality, more attention has recently focused on strategies avoiding bleeding complications.[21] Despite the development of new, more potent, selective, and safe antithrombotics, the use of TRA is probably the best method to significantly decrease access site–related bleeding risk.[22–25]

Recently, the REAL (Registro Regionale Angioplastiche dell'Emilia-Romagna) Registry of 11,068 patients with STEMI undergoing PPCI showed that TRA was associated with a decreased 2-year mortality compared with the traditional TFA (8.8% vs 11.4%, hazard ratio [HR], 1.303; P = .025).[12] The observed difference in death was not explained by the incidence of MI or stroke, which did not differ between groups. By contrast, TRA was associated with a significant and marked reduction of in-hospital major bleeding or vascular events.

The available clinical evidence summarized in recent meta-analyses showed a significant reduction in mortality, major adverse cardiac events (MACE), major bleeding events, and major access-site complications associated with the TRA.[24–26]

Therefore, the use of TRA for high-risk patients with STEMI has a key role in the prevention of access-site bleeding complications.[27]

RANDOMIZED TRIALS AND REGISTRIES OF TRANSRADIAL ACCESS VERSUS TRANSFEMORAL ACCESS IN PRIMARY PERCUTANEOUS CORONARY INTERVENTION

The RIVAL (Radial Versus Femoral Access for Coronary Angiography and Intervention in Patients with Acute Coronary Syndromes) is the largest randomized comparison of radial and femoral artery access, involving 7021 patients with ACS; 1958 with a prerandomization diagnosis of STEMI and 5063 patients with NSTEACS.[11] In patients with STEMI, TRA significantly reduced the primary outcome: death, MI, stroke or non–coronary artery bypass grafting–related major bleeding within 30 days (3.1% vs 5.2%; HR, 0.60; P = .026) and mortality alone (1.3% vs 3.2%; HR, 0.39; P = .006). In patients presenting with NSTEACS, there were no significant differences in any of these outcomes. In patients with STEMI and patients with NSTEACS, TRA reduced major vascular access-site complications (1.4% vs 3.7%; HR, 0.37; P<.0001) and major bleeding as defined by the Acute Catheterization and Urgent Intervention Triage strategY (ACUITY) definition (1.9% vs 4.5%; HR, 043; P<.0001). In patients with STEMI, the reductions in the primary and secondary composite outcomes were driven mainly by a reduction in mortality with a directionally consistent reduction in MI. No such benefit was observed in patients with NSTEACS. Access-site crossover was higher in the radial group compared with the femoral group (7.6% vs 2.0%; HR, 3.82; P<.0001), and this was consistent in both STEMI and NSTEACS cohorts.[28]

The RIFLE-STEACS (Radial Versus Femoral Investigation in ST Elevation Acute Coronary Syndrome) is the first large randomized clinical trial, with 1001 patients with STEMI specifically designed to compare the radial (500 patients) and femoral (501 patients) approaches for primary/rescue PCI. In this nearly all-comers study, TRA was associated with significantly lower rates of clinically relevant access-site bleeding (2.6% vs 6.8%; P = .002) and subsequent 30-day mortality (5.2% vs 9.2%; P = .020) compared with TFA. The reduction in cardiac mortality and clinically relevant access-site bleeding by 60% and a significant decrease in the need for transfusion in the radial arm of the RIFLE-STEACS support the link between mortality and clinically relevant access-site bleeding. Furthermore, there were no differences in the symptom-to-balloon and door-to-balloon times between the two study groups. Vascular approach crossover was

9.6% in the radial arm and 2.8% in the femoral arm, with negligible time delay with expert operators.[13]

Recently, the randomized STEMI-RADIAL (A Prospective Randomized Trial of Radial vs Femoral Access in Patients with ST Segment Elevation Myocardial Infarction) trial, showed that TRA was associated with a significantly lower incidence of major bleeding and access-site complications and a significantly better net clinical benefit composite of death, MI and stroke, and major bleeding (4.6% vs 11%; P = .0028) Moreover, TRA significantly reduced intensive coronary care unit stay (P = .0016) and contrast volume (P<.01) compared with TFA (Table 1).[29]

The post hoc analysis of the HORIZON-AMI (Harmonizing Outcomes With Revascularization and Stents in Acute Myocardial Infarction)[22] trial showed improved event-free survival in patients undergoing PPCI by the TRA and also confirmed the advantage of the TRA with regard to hemorrhagic complications in patients treated with bivalirudin.

Based on data derived from the RIFLE-STEACS and STEMI subgroup of RIVAL, in the latest 2012 European Society of Cardiology STEMI guideline recommendations, TRA is preferred to TFA if performed by an experienced operator (class IIa, level B).[30]

A recent meta-analysis of 12 randomized controlled studies involving 5055 patients showed a significant reduction in mortality with TRA, with the odds of death being almost one-half those for the TFA arm (odds ratio [OR], 0.55; 95% CI, 0.40–0.76; P<.001). A similar reduction was seen in the rate of major bleeding: 32 of 2308 (1.4%) versus 70 of 2377 (2.9%) (OR, 0.51; 95% CI, 0.31–0.85; P<.05) (Table 2).

Similarly, analysis of the North American National Cardiovascular Data Registry Cath-PCI registry, which included 90,879 patients who underwent either primary or rescue PCI for STEMI, showed that TRA was independently associated with reduction of in-hospital mortality (OR, 0.76; 95% CI, 0.57–0.99) and of bleeding (OR, 0.62; 95% CI, 0.53–0.72).[31]

Recently, single-center registry of 1808 consecutive all-comer patients with STEMI showed that complete transitioning from TFA to preferred TRA is safe and effective for PPCI with favorable short-term and long-term outcomes. Compared with TFA, the TRA was associated with lower cardiovascular mortality at 30 days and 1 year (5.2% vs 10.5%; OR, 0.46; 95% CI, 0.32–0.66; P<.001; and 6.9% vs 11.5%; OR, 0.57; 95% CI, 0.41–0.79; P = .01).[32]

In addition, the analysis of 46,128 PPCI cases recorded in the British Cardiovascular Intervention Society database over a 5-year period suggested that TRA was independently associated with a lower 30-day mortality (HR, 0.71; P<.05), in-hospital major adverse cardiac and cardiovascular events (MACCE) (HR, 0.73; P<.05), major bleeding (HR, 0.37; P<.01), and access-site complications (HR, 0.38; P<.01).[33]

Table 1
Summary of major randomized clinical trials comparing TRI and TFI

	Trial		
	RIVAL (N = 7021)	RIFLE-STEACS (N = 1001)	STEMI-RADIAL (N = 707)
Patients, TRI/TFI (n)	3507/3514	500/501	348/359
Type of patients	ACS: STEMI, 27.9% NSTEMI, 27.1% UA, 45%	STEMI	STEMI
Heparin (IU/kg)	NA	70/71	103/105
GP IIb/IIIa inhibitors (%)	25.3/24.0	67.4/69.9	15/15
Bivalirudin (%)	2.2/3.1	8.0/7.2	NA
Catheter ≤6 F (%)	91.8/87.0	90.8/81.4	100/99.8
Major bleeding (%)	0.8/0.9 (P = .87)	7.8/12.2 (P = .026)	1.4/11.0 (P = .0001)
MACE (%)	2.7/4.6 (P = .031)	7.2/11.4 (P = .029)	3.5/4.2 (P = .7)
Mortality (%)	1.3/3.2 (P = .006)	5.2/9.2 (P = .02)	2.3/3.1 (P = .64)

Abbreviations: GP, glycoprotein; NA, data not available; NSTEMI, non–ST segment elevation myocardial infarction; RIFLE-STEACS, Radial Versus Femoral Randomized Investigation in ST Elevation Acute Coronary Syndrome trial; RIVAL, Radial Versus Femoral Access for Coronary Intervention; STEMI-RADIAL, ST Elevation Myocardial infarction Treated by Radial or Femoral Approach – Randomized Multicenter Study Comparing Radial Versus Femoral Approach in Primary PCI trial; TFI, transfemoral intervention; TRI, transradial intervention; UA, unstable angina.

Table 2 Radial versus femoral approach in STEMI: a meta-analysis of 12 randomized controlled studies			
	Radial	Femoral	P Value
Mortality (%)	2.7	4.7	<.001 ↓
Major bleeding (%)	1.4	2.9	.01 ↓
Access-site bleeding (%)	2.1	5.6	<.001 ↓
Stroke (%)	0.5	0.5	.87
Procedure time mean difference (min)		1.52	

N = 5055 patients.
Data from Karrowni W, Vyas A, Giacomino B, et al. Radial versus femoral access for primary percutaneous interventions in ST-segment elevation myocardial infarction patients. A meta-analysis of randomized controlled trials. JACC Cardiovasc Interv 2013;6:814–23.

However, the 0.7% absolute reduction in major bleeding and 0.3% absolute reduction in access site–related complications associated with TRA use cannot fully explain the scale of the mortality benefit associated with TRA in PPCI[33]

Additional unmeasured factors may contribute to the benefit of TRA PPCI.

Although some access-site complications do not result in significant blood loss, they may lead to systemic inflammation, activation of prothrombotic pathways, and activation of the clotting cascade. This outcome could further increase the risk of cardiovascular events even though the initial insult is not hemodynamically significant.[34,35]

Bleeding or access-site complications can also lead to withdrawal of antiplatelet agents, increasing the risk of ischemic complications (Fig. 1).

HIGH-RISK SUBGROUPS FOR BLEEDING AND VASCULAR COMPLICATIONS

Patients undergoing PCI in the context of STEMI are expected to receive a combination of potent multiple antithrombotic drugs that may lead to an increased risk of bleeding and subsequent morbidity and mortality.

Women are at higher risk of bleeding and other adverse outcomes after PCI than men.[36,37] In a recent observational study, routine TRA was associated with reduced bleeding risk in women.[38] However, muscular arterial hyperreactivity, procedural discomfort, and small artery diameter increases the risk of first radial access failure (9.6% in women vs 1.6% in men). However, successful radial access does not allow the operator to use more aggressive combinations of anticoagulants and antiplatelet agents in this group, given that women remain at higher non–access-site bleeding risk.[39,40]

Elderly patients are also at high risk for bleeding and vascular complications after PCI. Lower limb peripheral artery disease (PAD), tortuosity of the iliac arteries, and aneurysms of the abdominal aorta may represent relative or absolute contraindications to TFA. Because of PAD in the elderly, radial access seems to be as feasible

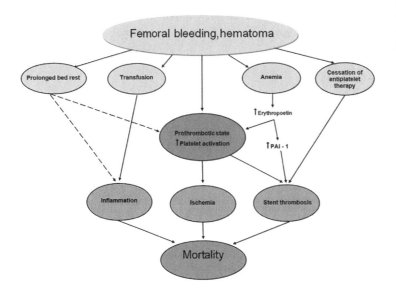

Fig. 1. Hypothetical mechanisms linking femoral bleeding with excess mortality. PAI-1, plasminogen activator inhibitor.

as femoral access. In 2 randomized trials, the TRA was associated with fewer vascular complications in elderly patients.[41,42]

ST SEGMENT ELEVATION MYOCARDIAL INFARCTION PRESENTING WITH CARDIOGENIC SHOCK

Cardiogenic shock has poor outcomes compared with less severe presentations of STEMI.

The SHOCK (Should We Emergently Revascularize Occluded Coronaries for Cardiogenic Shock) trial[42] showed the importance of revascularization to improve outcomes, but the recent IABP-SHOCK II Trial[43] failed to show any marginal benefit of adding hemodynamic support with intra-aortic balloon (IABP) counterpulsation in the setting of shock.

Cardiogenic shock is associated with a doubling of the risk of bleeding compared with the absence of shock.[44] There may be a safety advantage in using the radial artery for the coronary intervention and reserving the femoral artery for larger devices in patients with cardiogenic shock.

Rodriguez-Leor and colleagues[45] analyzed their single-center registry experience with radial access in patients with cardiogenic shock. From 1400-patients, 122 (8.7%) developed cardiogenic shock, with 80 undergoing transfemoral catheterization and the remaining 42 undergoing transradial catheterization. Mortality (64.3% vs 32.5%; P<.001), serious access-site complications (11.9% vs 2.5%; P<.03), access-site complications requiring blood transfusion (7.1% vs 0%; P<.04), and MACCE (death, infarction, stroke, serious bleeding, and postanoxic encephalopathy) (73.8% vs 43.8%; P<.001) were greater in patients treated by the femoral route. After multivariate analysis, initial TRA was associated with lower mortality (OR, 0.39 [0.15–0.97]) compared with an initial TFA.[45]

Bernat and colleagues[46] evaluated the outcomes of 197 patients with STEMI with signs of cardiogenic shock who were treated with PPCI at 2 high-volume centers. The TRA was used successfully in 55% of cases in which at least 1 radial artery was weakly palpable. TRA emerged as independent predictor of survival, with more than half patients treated successfully. Mortality at 1 year was 44% in the radial group and 64% in the femoral group (P = .0044).

Romagnoli and colleagues[47] analyzed 241 consecutive patients (91% with ACS and left main culprit in 26% of cases) receiving IABP support during PCI in 4 high-volume centers. Patients were further divided into 2 groups: 116 patients receiving double femoral access (FF)

and 125 patients receiving both radial and femoral (RF) approaches. Net adverse clinical events (NACEs) were more frequent in the FF group compared with the RF group (67% vs 41%; P<.01). In particular, this difference originated from an increase of access site–related bleeding (21% vs 7%; P<.01) and cardiac death (41% vs 25%; P<.01).

These data show that an FR access strategy is safer than a FF access strategy, and that this safety advantage is associated with reduced mortality.[47]

A significant involvement of the left main coronary artery occurs in 4% to 7% of patients presenting with STEMI.[48,49] These critically ill patients frequently present with cardiogenic shock or cardiac arrest and are at high risk for in-hospital MACEs.[50,51]

STEMI PPCI because of a unprotected left main coronary artery (ULMCA) culprit lesion is a rare procedure, frequently associated with adverse clinical outcomes. The incidence of STEMI of a ULMCA culprit lesion is reported to be 0.8% to 5.4%.[52]

Patients undergoing STEMI PPCI because of a ULMCA culprit lesion and presenting with cardiogenic shock have high 30-day mortality compared with patients without cardiogenic shock, with an estimated 30-day all-cause mortality of 55% for patients with cardiogenic shock and 15% for patients without cardiogenic shock.

Most PCIs in high-risk patients with STEMI can be performed by TRA through conventional 6-F guiding catheters, including complex cases, those with left main bifurcations, and those with cardiogenic shock. However, a stepwise approach to learning and high-risk STEMI PCI is recommended as the last step (Fig. 2).

The treatment of patients in shock requires an individualized approach. Although the radial pulse may return with vasopressor administration, there may be clinical situations in which radial access is not possible and femoral access must be used. From the available evidence supporting the safety of the TRA rather than TFA, a radial-first strategy likely still applies in most patients, even those with large STEMI and shock if performed by skilled and experienced radial operators. Hemodynamic support devices can be placed via the femoral route and temporary pacemakers can be placed through forearm or femoral veins.[53]

ULNAR ARTERY ACCESS

The TRA may be difficult or associated with increased risk of complications in the presence of significant radial artery abnormalities, severe loops and curvatures, after failed radial artery

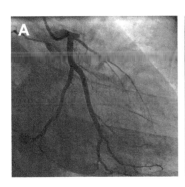
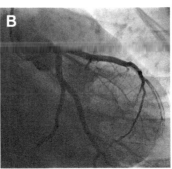

Fig. 2. PPCI in anterior wall STEMI. (A) Proximal left anterior descending artery occlusion. (B) Result after PPCI with bioresorbable vascular scaffold (BVS) 3.5/18 mm under optical coherence tomography guidance.

cannulation, and when the radial artery was repeatedly used previously.

Transulnar artery cannulation (TUA) has been proposed as an alternative access for interventions in patients with small-caliber radial artery or thin radial pulse and stronger pulsation of the ulnar artery. Larger studies have further confirmed the safety and effectiveness of TUA as an alternative wrist approach to TRA for coronary interventions.[16,54]

The procedural success, advantages, and complication rates for transulnar interventions seem to be similar to those of TRA.[15,54] Adding expertise in ulnar artery access could further reduce the crossover rate to TFA and reduce the intrinsic risk of bleeding and vascular complications associated with TFA. When TRA is not possible or fails, TUA may be considered as a safe alternative before reverting to TFA.[16] TUA is a viable option for high-volume radial centers when performed by expert radial operators who are skilled in ulnar artery cannulation.[54]

LIMITATIONS OF THE TRANSRADIAL ACCESS FOR COMPLEX PRIMARY PERCUTANEOUS CORONARY INTERVENTION

Longer procedure duration and radiation exposure during the learning curve and the potential influence on radial artery patency have slowed acceptance of the TRA. The technique of TRA requires a specific set of skills and is associated with a significant learning curve. With appropriate training, similar success rates with TRA and TFA may be achieved even in complex STEMI cases. The learning curve is highly individual and more experienced operators may become proficient sooner.

To achieve the best results in TRA interventions, individual operators and institutional teams should try to maintain the highest feasible rate of TRA. After the learning curve has been completed, for more than 50% of TRA in routine practice, a minimum of 80 procedures per year per operator are recommended.[55]

A stepwise approach to learning is proposed according to clinical characteristics and PCI difficulty. PPCI in STEMI is proposed as the last step because of multifaceted clinical settings and PCI complexity. The highest level of competency is obtained when complex PPCI can be performed in a timely and technically proficient manner irrespective of vascular access anatomy.[55]

TRA is associated with a low incidence (0.2%) of major vascular complications.[10] Hematomas are usually minor, affecting only subcutaneous tissue. Unlike groin bleeding, subcutaneous bleeding after TRA is rapidly noticed and can be controlled by local compression. Major vascular complications like compartment syndrome are almost completely avoidable.

Radial artery occlusion (RAO) is the most common complication, affecting 1.5% to 33% of patients shortly after the procedure, depending on the antithrombotic regimen, sheath size, and protocol for haemostasis.[56] Although usually asymptomatic, RAO is an important consequence of TRA, because it prohibits future ipsilateral TRA. Preserving radial artery patency is of paramount importance. Proper anticoagulation, downsizing of material (slender sheaths and sheathless catheters), and shorter and less forceful patent hemostasis of the radial artery, with the emphasis on maintaining adequate arterial flow, considerably reduces the risk of RAO.

It is important to remember that almost all potential complications are preventable by accurate preprocedural evaluation, meticulous technique, and optimal postprocedural management.

The incidence of RAS has varied considerably (4%–30%) depending on its definition, study population, and the expertise of the operators.[55] Spasm is the second most common cause of radial access failure after anatomic variations. The incidence of moderate/severe RAS is low in centers with default TRA (2.7%). Its development and procedural failure (0.7%) seem to be strongly related to the numbers of puncture attempts and the use of larger-bore sheaths.[57]

TECHNICAL RECOMMENDATIONS FOR TRANSRADIAL ACCESS PRIMARY PERCUTANEOUS CORONARY INTERVENTION

There should be previous experience with TRA and diagnostics and elective PCI in approximately 100 cases, with TFA crossover less than 4%. Success of TRA PPCI depends almost entirely on the catheter laboratory staff.

At the beginning of the learning curve, challenging anatomy must be avoided to minimize the risk of complications and shorten the duration of both the procedure and radiation exposure. For this reason, a systematic preliminary angiogram of the forearm arteries through the radial introducer or long cannula is highly recommended. Highly tortuous and spasmatic RA segments could be crossed with PCI guidewire and exchanged with 0.889-mm (0.035-inch) guidewire over a small-caliber (4-F or 5-F) diagnostic catheter (Fig. 3 and Videos 1 and 2).

The eventual choice of procedure depends on operator's expertise and the equipment required. The right side is usually more ergonomic to the operator; however, the left TRA might be more convenient in the learning phase because of similar catheter handling compared with the TFA.

Even if dedicated catheter shapes are available, traditional femoral shapes accommodate the radial approach easily. Coaxial alignment with the target coronary artery is mandatory and requires different handling for the right radial versus femoral approach.

The choice of guiding catheter (diameter, shape, size) is essential for adequate backup. A buddy wire in the non–infarct-related artery might be considered to improve guiding catheter stability.

Most PCIs can be performed through 6-F guiding catheters, including complex cases, thrombus aspiration, after CABG, and left main bifurcations (Fig. 4).

In selected patients, large-lumen guiding catheters (7 F) advanced with a mother-and-child technique can be considered. Sheathless guiding catheters are useful in selected cases, but are more difficult to handle in complex procedures because there is less backup.

In patients with cardiogenic shock, TRA procedures can be performed if the radial artery is palpable while leaving 2 potential femoral

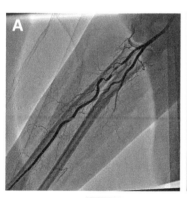
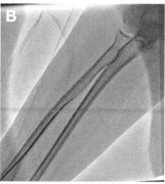
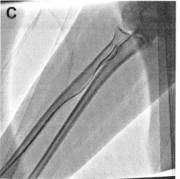

Fig. 3. Right forearm angiogram with significant tortuosity and spasm of radial artery. (A) Tortuous and spasmatic radial artery. (B) PCI wire advancement. (C) 5-F Judkins right (JR) diagnostic catheter advancement.

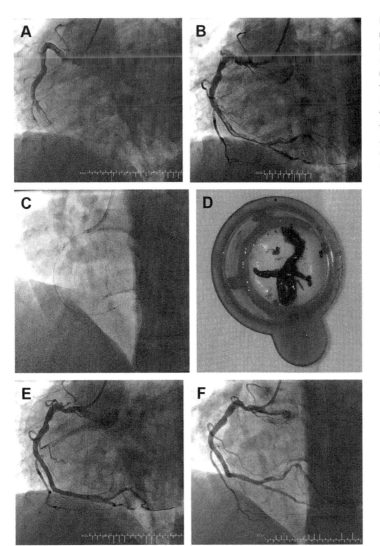

Fig. 4. PPCI of highly thrombotic mid-right coronary artery (mid-RCA) occlusion. (A) Complete thrombotic occlusion of mid-RCA. (B) Result after wiring with large thrombus propagation. (C) Repetitive manual thromboaspiration with 6-F catheter. (D) Large thrombus retrieval. (E) Result after drug eluting stent (DES) (3.5/15 mm) at mid-RCA. (F) Final result.

accesses for IABP counterpulsation or more complex cardiac-assist devices.

RAO should be prevented during and after the procedure with systematic assessment of the arterial patency.[58]

Spasm prevention with 3 to 5 mg of verapamil administered intra-arterially through the sheath is recommended routinely. Specific early and delayed postprocedural attention to forearm hematomas is mandatory.

SUMMARY

There is significant evidence supporting a shift to a preferred TRA for most PPCI procedures with an emphasis on decreasing access-site bleeding and vascular complications without compromising procedural outcome. Systematic use of TRA is probably the best mode to significantly decrease access site–related bleeding risk. A high-risk subset of patients with complex STEMI for bleeding and vascular complications such as in women and the elderly might particularly benefit from TRA whenever appropriately available and performed by skilled operators.

Complications arising from TRA are infrequent, negligible, and mostly avoidable compared with TFA complications. Certain limitations to TRA, such as longer radiation exposure during the learning curve and the potential influence on radial artery patency, have slowed acceptance of this technique. Modern interventional cardiologists should go through a high-volume radial training program after developing the optimal radial experience to adopt the TRA first whenever possible.

Adding ulnar artery access expertise could further reduce the crossover rate to TFA and reduce the intrinsic risk of bleeding and vascular complications associated with TFA. The femoral approach is likely to remain a viable alternative for patients not eligible for the wrist access and accessory access for larger devices in patients with cardiogenic shock.

Only experienced high-volume radialists should perform complex PPCIs in patients with cardiogenic shock and left main culprit.

In addition, selection of an access site is only one part of improving patients' outcomes. All interventions should be performed according to the highest available standards, ensuring the best treatment of each patient without compromising procedural success and long-term prognosis.

SUPPLEMENTARY DATA

Supplementary data related to this article can be found online at http://dx.doi.org/10.1016/j.iccl.2014.12.003.

REFERENCES

1. Keeley EC, Boura JA, Grines CL. Primary angioplasty versus intra-venous thrombolytic therapy for acute myocardial infarction: a quantitative review of 23 randomised trials. Lancet 2003;361:13–20.

2. Mehta SR, Cannon CP, Fox KA, et al. Routine vs selective invasive strategies in patients with acute coronary syndromes: a collaborative meta-analysis of randomized trials. JAMA 2005;293:2908–17.

3. Doyle BJ, Ting HH, Bell MR, et al. Major femoral bleeding complications after percutaneous coronary intervention: incidence, predictors, and impact on long-term survival among 17,901 patients treated at the Mayo Clinic from 1994 to 2005. JACC Cardiovasc Interv 2008;1:202–9.

4. Elbarouni B, Elmanfud O, Yan RT, et al. Temporal trend of in-hospital major bleeding among patients with non ST-elevation acute coronary syndromes. Am Heart J 2010;160:420–7.

5. Steg PG, Huber K, Andreotti F, et al. Bleeding in acute coronary syndromes and percutaneous coronary interventions: position paper by the Working Group on Thrombosis of the European Society of Cardiology. Eur Heart J 2011;32:1854–64.

6. Mehran R, Pocock SJ, Stone GW, et al. Associations of major bleeding and myocardial infarction with the incidence and timing of mortality in patients presenting with non-ST-elevation acute coronary syndromes: a risk model from the ACUITY trial. Eur Heart J 2009;30:1457–66.

7. Campeau L. Percutaneous radial artery approach for coronary angiography. Cathet Cardiovasc Diagn 1989;16:3–7.

8. Kiemeneij F, Laarman GJ. Percutaneous transradial artery approach for coronary stent implantation. Cathet Cardiovasc Diagn 1993;30:173–8.

9. Rao SV, Ou FS, Wang TY, et al. Trends in the prevalence and outcomes of radial and femoral approaches to percutaneous coronary intervention: a report from the National Cardiovascular Data Registry. JACC Cardiovasc Interv 2008;1:379–86.

10. Kiemeneij F, Laarman GJ, Odekerken D, et al. A randomized comparison of percutaneous transluminal coronary angioplasty by the radial, brachial and femoral approaches: the access study. J Am Coll Cardiol 1997;29:1269–75.

11. Jolly SS, Yusuf S, Cairns J, et al, RIVAL Trial Group. Radial versus femoral access for coronary angiography and intervention in patients with acute coronary syndromes (RIVAL): a randomised, parallel group, multicentre trial. Lancet 2011;377:1409–20.

12. Valgimigli M, Saia F, Guastaroba P, et al. Transradial versus transfemoral intervention for acute myocardial infarction. A propensity score-adjusted and -matched analysis from the REAL (REgistro regionale AngiopLastiche dell'Emilia-Romagna) multicenter registry. JACC Cardiovasc Interv 2012; 5:23–35.

13. Romagnoli E, Biondi-Zoccai G, Sciahbasi A, et al. Radial versus femoral randomized investigation in ST-segment elevation acute coronary syndrome: the RIFLE-STEACS (Radial Versus Femoral Randomized Investigation in ST-Elevation Acute Coronary Syndrome) study. J Am Coll Cardiol 2012;60:2481–9.

14. Vink MA, Amoroso G, Dirksen MT, et al. Routine use of the transradial approach in primary percutaneous coronary intervention: procedural aspects and outcomes in 2209 patients treated in a single high-volume centre. Heart 2011;97:1938–42.

15. Kedev S. Transulnar approach: pros and cons. In: Patel T, editor. Patel's atlas of transradial intervention the basics and beyond. Malvern (PA): HMP Communications; 2012. p. 221–32.

16. Andrade PB, Tebet MA, Nogueira EF, et al. Transulnar approach as an alternative access site for coronary invasive procedures after transradial approach failure. Am Heart J 2012;164:462–7.

17. Fuchs S, Kornowski R, Teplitsky I, et al. Major bleeding complicating contemporary primary percutaneous coronary interventions — incidence, predictors, and prognostic implications. Cardiovasc Revasc Med 2009;10:88–93.

18. Applegate RJ, Sacrinty MT, Kutcher MA, et al. Trends in vascular complications after diagnostic cardiac catheterization and percutaneous coronary intervention via the femoral artery, 1998 to 2007. JACC Cardiovasc Interv 2008;1:317–26.

19. Verheugt FW, Steinhubl SR, Hamon M, et al. Incidence, prognostic impact, and influence of antithrombotic therapy on access and non-access site bleeding in percutaneous coronary intervention. JACC Cardiovasc Interv 2011;4:191 7.

20. Hermanides RS, Ottervanger JP, Dambrink JH, et al. Incidence, predictors and prognostic importance of bleeding after primary PCI for ST-elevation myocardial infarction. EuroIntervention 2010;6:106–11.

21. Budaj A, Eikelboom JW, Mehta SR, et al. Improving clinical outcomes by reducing bleeding in patients with non-ST-elevation acute coronary syndromes. Eur Heart J 2009;30:655–61.

22. Généreux P, Mehran R, Palmerini T, et al, HORIZONS-AMI Trial Investigators. Radial access in patients with ST-segment elevation myocardial infarction undergoing primary angioplasty in acute myocardial infarction: the HORIZONS-AMI trial. EuroIntervention 2011;7:905–16.

23. Jolly SS, Amlani S, Hamon M, et al. Radial versus femoral access for coronary angiography or intervention and the impact on major bleeding and ischemic events: a systematic review and meta-analysis of randomized trials. Am Heart J 2009; 157:132–40.

24. Mamas MA, Ratib K, Routledge H, et al. Influence of access site selection on PCI-related adverse events in patients with STEMI: meta-analysis of randomised controlled trials. Heart 2012;98:303–11.

25. Bertrand OF, Bélisle P, Joyal D, et al. Comparison of transradial and femoral approaches for percutaneous coronary interventions: a systematic review and hierarchical Bayesian meta-analysis. Am Heart J 2012;163:632–48.

26. Karrowni W, Vyas A, Giacomino B, et al. Radial versus femoral access for primary percutaneous interventions in ST-segment elevation myocardial infarction patients. A meta-analysis of randomized controlled trials. JACC Cardiovasc Interv 2013;6: 814–23.

27. Rao SV, Cohen MG, Kandzari DE, et al. The transradial approach to percutaneous coronary intervention: historical perspective, current concepts, and future directions. J Am Coll Cardiol 2010;55:2187–95.

28. Mehta SR, Jolly SS, Cairns J, et al, RIVAL Investigators. Effects of radial versus femoral artery access in patients with acute coronary syndromes with or without ST-segment elevation. J Am Coll Cardiol 2012;60(24):2490–9.

29. Bernat I, Horak D, Stasek J, et al. ST-segment elevation myocardial infarction treated by radial or femoral approach in a multicenter randomized clinical trial: the STEMI-RADIAL trial. J Am Coll Cardiol 2014;63:964–72.

30. Steg PG, James SK, Task Force on the management of ST-segment elevation acute myocardial infarction of the European Society of Cardiology (ESC). ESC guidelines for the management of acute myocardial infarction in patients presenting with ST-segment elevation. Eur Heart J 2012;33:2569–619.

31. Baklanov DV, Kaltenbach LA, Marso SP, et al. The prevalence and outcomes of transradial percutaneous coronary intervention for ST-segment elevation myocardial infarction: analysis from the National Cardiovascular Data Registry (2007 to 2011). J Am Coll Cardiol 2013;61:420–6.

32. Kedev S, Kalpak O, Dharma S, et al. Complete transitioning to the radial approach for primary percutaneous coronary intervention: a real-world single-center registry of 1808 consecutive patients with acute ST-elevation myocardial infarction. J Invasive Cardiol 2014;26(9):475–82.

33. Mamas AM, Ratib K, Routledge H, et al. Influence of arterial access site selection on outcomes in primary percutaneous coronary intervention: are the results of randomized trials achievable in clinical practice? JACC Cardiovasc Interv 2013;6:698–706.

34. Doyle BJ, Rihal CS, Gastineau DA, et al. Bleeding, blood transfusion, and increased mortality after percutaneous coronary intervention. Implications for contemporary practice. J Am Coll Cardiol 2009;53:2019–27.

35. Allen C, Glasziou P, Del Mar C. Bed rest: a potentially harmful treatment needing more careful evaluation. Lancet 1999;354:1229–33.

36. Chauhan MS, Ho KK, Baim DS, et al. Effect of gender on in-hospital and one-year outcomes after contemporary coronary artery stenting. Am J Cardiol 2005;95:101–4.

37. Nikolsky E, Mehran R, Dangas G, et al. Development and validation of a prognostic risk score for major bleeding in patients undergoing percutaneous coronary intervention via the femoral approach. Eur Heart J 2007;28:1936–45.

38. Pristipino C, Pelliccia F, Granatelli A, et al. Comparison of access-related bleeding complications in women versus men undergoing percutaneous coronary catheterization using the radial versus femoral artery. Am J Cardiol 2007;99:1216–21.

39. Valsecchi O, Musumeci G, Vassileva A, et al. Safety and feasibility of transradial coronary angioplasty in elderly patients. Ital Heart J 2004;5:926–31.

40. Louvard Y, Benamer H, Garot P, et al. Comparison of transradial and transfemoral approaches for coronary angiography and angioplasty in octogenarians (the OCTOPLUS study). Am J Cardiol 2004; 94:1177–80.

41. Achenbach S, Ropers D, Kallert L, et al. Transradial versus transfemoral approach for coronary angiography and intervention in patients above 75 years of age. Catheter Cardiovasc Interv 2008;72:629–35.

42. Hochman JS, Sleeper LA, Webb JG, et al. Early revascularization in acute myocardial infarction

complicated by cardiogenic shock. SHOCK Investigators. Should we emergently revascularize occluded coronaries for cardiogenic shock. N Engl J Med 1999;341:625–34.

43. Thiele H, Zeymer U, Neumann FJ, et al. Intraaortic balloon support for myocardial infarction with cardiogenic shock. N Engl J Med 2012;367:1287–96.

44. Mehta SK, Frutkin AD, Lindsey JB, et al. Bleeding in patients undergoing percutaneous coronary intervention: the development of a clinical risk algorithm from the National Cardiovascular Data Registry. Circ Cardiovasc Interv 2009;2:222–9.

45. Rodriguez-Leor O, Fernandez-Nofrerias E, Carrillo X, et al. Transradial percutaneous coronary intervention in cardiogenic shock: a single-center experience. Am Heart J 2013;165:280–5.

46. Bernat I, Abdelaal E, Plourde G, et al. Early and late outcomes after primary percutaneous coronary intervention by radial or femoral approach in patients presenting in acute ST-elevation myocardial infarction and cardiogenic shock. Am Heart J 2013;165(3):338–43.

47. Romagnoli E, De Vita M, Burzotta F, et al. Clinical benefit of radial versus femoral approach in percutaneous coronary intervention with intra-aortic balloon pump support. J Am Coll Cardiol 2012;60(17 Suppl):B9–10.

48. Goldberg S, Grossman W, Markis JE, et al. Total occlusion of the left main coronary artery. A clinical, hemodynamic and angiographic profile. Am J Med 1978;64:3–8.

49. Spiecker M, Erbel R, Rupprecht HJ, et al. Emergency angioplasty of totally occluded left main coronary artery in acute myocardial infarction and unstable angina pectoris—institutional experience and literature review. Eur Heart J 1994;15:602–7.

50. de Feyter PJ, Serruys PW. Thrombolysis of acute total occlusion of the left main coronary artery in evolving myocardial infarction. Am J Cardiol 1984;53:1727–8.

51. Quigley RL, Milano CA, Smith LR, et al. Prognosis and management of anterolateral myocardial infarction in patients with severe left main disease and cardiogenic shock. The left main shock syndrome. Circulation 1993;88:II65–70.

52. Vis MM, Beijk MA, Grundeken MJ, et al. A systematic review and meta-analysis on primary percutaneous coronary intervention of an unprotected left main coronary artery culprit lesion in the setting of acute myocardial infarction. JACC Cardiovasc Interv 2013;6:317–24.

53. Gilchrist IC, Sunil V, Rao SV. Improving outcomes in patients with cardiogenic shock. Achieving more through less. Am Heart J 2013;165(3):256–7.

54. Kedev S, Zafirovska B, Surya Dharma S, et al. Safety and feasibility of transulnar catheterization when ipsilateral radial access is not available. Catheter Cardiovasc Interv 2014;83:E51–60.

55. Hamon M, Pristipino C, Di Mario C, et al. Consensus document on the radial approach in percutaneous cardiovascular interventions: position paper by the EAPCI and working groups on acute cardiac care and thrombosis of the European Society of Cardiology. EuroIntervention 2013;8:1242–51.

56. Geijer H, Persliden J. Radiation exposure and patient experience during percutaneous coronary intervention using radial and femoral artery access. Eur Radiol 2004;14:1674–80.

57. Goldsmit A, Kiemeneij F, Gilchrist IC, et al. Radial artery spasm associated with transradial cardiovascular procedures: results from the RAS registry. Catheter Cardiovasc Interv 2014;83:E32–6.

58. Pancholy SB, Patel TM. Effect of duration of hemostatic compression on radial artery occlusion after transradial access. Catheter Cardiovasc Interv 2012;79:78–81.

Transradial Peripheral Arterial Procedures

Kintur Sanghvi, MD, FSCAI[a,b,*], John Coppola, MD, FSCAI[c]

KEYWORDS

- Transradial catheterization • Radial approach for peripheral artery disease • Transradial endovascular interventions • Carotid artery intervention • Subclavian artery intervention • Renal artery intervention • Iliac artery intervention • Superficial femoral artery intervention

---

KEY POINTS

- Advantages of the transradial approach include less bleeding and other access-related complications, early ambulation and discharge, cost savings, and patient preference.
- Major limitations of the radial approach for peripheral interventions is lack of dedicated equipment with adequate working shaft length and smaller outer diameter.
- Multiple case series and technical reports exist showing the feasibility of the radial approach for treatment of different endovascular lesions from subclavian, carotid, abdominal arteries and lower extremity vessels.

Videos of transradial peripheral arterial procedures accompany this article at http://www.interventional.theclinics.com/

INTRODUCTION

In 2014, the debate over the safety and efficacy of transradial (TR) approach for cardiac catheterization is over. Reduced bleeding and other access-related complications, early ambulation and discharge, cost savings, and patient preference because of improved postprocedure comfort with faster recovery are some of the important reasons for the increased adoption of TR approach worldwide.[1-3] Because of the safety associated with radial access, the European Society of Cardiology consensus statement has recommended that radial access should be the default approach for cardiac catheterization.[3] A recent update using a retrospective cohort study from the CATH-PCI data registry showed an increase in TR interventions in the United States from 1.2% in the first quarter of

2007 to 16.1% in the third quarter of 2012, and may well be more than 20% at this time.[4]

In the presence of peripheral vascular disease (PVD), diagnostic and interventional cardiac catheterization procedures are associated with higher incidences of access-related complications.[5-7] A substudy of the CARP trial looked at 1298 patients with PVD undergoing diagnostic cardiac catheterization and showed a greater frequency of complications, including 22 major and 27 minor access-related complications.[8] In a retrospective review of 297 patients with aortofemoral PVD, upper extremity approaches for angiography were associated with lower complications compared with a femoral approach.[9]

The prevalence of peripheral artery disease in the United States is expected to grow from 8 to 12 million.[10,11] Percutaneous endovascular

---

There is no relevant disclosure for any conflict by either of the authors for the work here. No grant or sponsorship was received by either author for this work.
[a] Department of Interventional Cardiology and Endovascular Medicine, Deborah Heart & Lung Center, 200 Trenton Road, Browns Mills, NJ 08015, USA; [b] Philadelphia College of Osteopathic Medicine, Philadelphia, PA 19131, USA; [c] Department of Cardiology, NYU Langone Medical Center, 550 1st Avenue, New York, NY 10016, USA
* Corresponding author.
E-mail address: kintur@yahoo.com

treatment of PVD is the fastest growing proce-dure.[11] The recognition of higher access-related bleeding complications in the presence of PVD and the demonstrated reduction in these complications by the TR approach have led to fresh interest in TR endovascular treatment of PVD. Multiple case series and technical reports exist showing the feasibility of the radial approach for treatment of different endovascu-lar lesions from subclavian, carotid, abdominal arteries and lower extremity vessels.

FROM RADIAL ARTERY TO THE ENDOVASCULAR TARGET: TIPS AND TRICKS FOR SAFE AND EFFICIENT ACCESS TO THE PERIPHERAL CIRCULATION
Using the Knowledge of Radial Artery Size and Sheath Size

- The outer diameter (OD) of a sheath is almost 2 French (Fr) larger than the OD of the guide catheter of the same Fr size. For example, a 6-Fr glide sheath (Terumo Corporation, Somerset, NJ) has an OD of 2.61 mm and the OD of a 6-Fr guide catheter is 2.0 mm.
- Females, patients with small body mass index, and those with a smaller wrist size are likely to have smaller radial artery (RA). Whenever a patient's RA seems to be small based on clinical characteristics and palpation of the RA, rather than inserting the entire length of the introducer sheath and stretching the RA, the operator can insert 1 cm of the sheath into the RA (Fig. 1). This maneuver provides an atraumatic entry of the guide

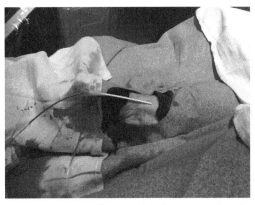

Fig. 1. Only 1 cm of a 7-Fr sheath is inserted in the radial artery to allow use of a 7-Fr guide catheter in a small size radial artery. (*From* Sanghvi K. Ten critical lessons for performing transradial catheterization. Endovascular Today 2014.)

in to RA; because the catheter has a smaller OD, it is less likely to expand the artery and cause irritation, spasm, or dissection of the RA. We often use 7-Fr guide catheters with this technique when the need to use a larger balloon-expandable stents arises (see Fig. 1).
- A similar understanding of the length and OD of long sheaths is equally important for TR endovascular intervention. The currently available long sheaths that were originally designed for femoral access (60, 90, 110 cm), have nearly 1 Fr larger OD than a short sheath of same Fr size and are more likely to cause spasm. A 6-Fr, 90-cm Destination sheath (Terumo Corporation, Somerset, NJ) has OD of 2.83 mm. The Destination sheath does not have hydrophilic coating on the entire length of the catheter.

Using the Knowledge of Distance From the Radial Artery and Equipment Length

- A major limitation of the RA approach for peripheral intervention is the lack of equipment with adequate shaft length to reach distal vascular lesions. Anthropometric measurement in Fig. 2 gives an approximate idea of the distance from the RA to different vascular beds.
- Using the right RA access for infradiaphragm vessels reduces operator radiation exposure, but left RA access increases the usable length of the catheter systems by about 10 cm.
- Positioning the patient supine in a reverse position (feet at the head end of the table) allows the operator to work from left RA easily, reach farther distal target in the lower extremity and reduces x-ray exposure (Fig. 3).
- When inadequate working shaft length is anticipated, the RA can be accessed 2 to 3 inches higher than normal; at this level, the RA is deeper but still separated from major nerves in the forearm. This high entry requires extra attention to hemostasis.
- The distances in Fig. 2 can vary depending on the extent of the tortuosity in the subclavian or brachiocephalic vessels, tortuosity and dilation of the aorta, and the height of the patient. By using a stiff wire inside the guide catheter when tortuosity is encountered, the tortuosity can be straightened, allowing the catheter

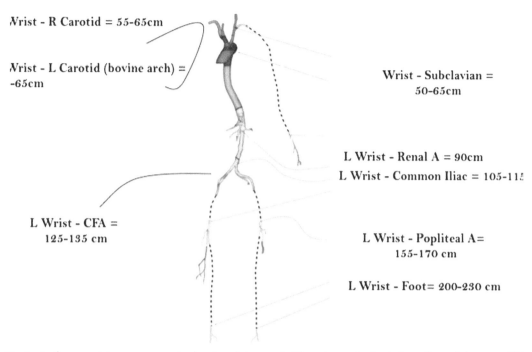

Wrist - R Carotid = 55-65cm

Wrist - L Carotid (bovine arch) = -65cm

Wrist - Subclavian = 50-65cm

L Wrist - Renal A = 90cm
L Wrist - Common Iliac = 105-11£

L Wrist - CFA = 125-135 cm

L Wrist - Popliteal A= 155-170 cm

L Wrist - Foot= 200-230 cm

Fig. 2. Anthropometric measurements showing distance of different vascular beds from the radial artery. CFA, common femoral artery; L, left; R, right.

to reach farther down the descending aorta. Table 1 includes a listing of the major available endovascular devices in the United States that can be used through a 6-Fr sheath and have working length adequate for TR use. The major advantage of using a 90- or 110-cm sheath is the ability to perform intermittent

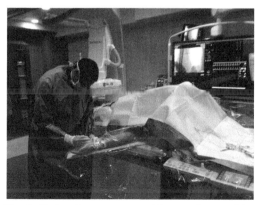

Fig. 3. Patient in a reverse position to allow working from the left radial artery for lower extremity interventions. Note that the x-ray source and image intensifier are away from the operator.

angiographic evaluation through the sheath to position a balloon or stents.

- An alternate method is to use a short sheath and a 125-cm-long guide catheter (Video 1.1; available online at http://www.interventional.theclinics.com/). In that instance, after defining the anatomy and crossing the lesion with a 300-cm-long support wire (0.035″ or 0.018″) the guide catheter is removed and the treatment devices are delivered over the guide wire using image overlay, radiopaque markers or bony landmarks (see Videos 1.2 and 1.3; available online at http://www.interventional.theclinics.com/). This approach should not be used when the RA is originating high from axillary or brachial artery because there is a potential risk of stent entrapment owing to severe spasm of the RA, recurrent RA, or accessory RA when a short sheath is used and the devices are deliver over long 0.035″ or 0.018″ wires.
- _Entering the descending aorta:_ A left anterior oblique 40° view opens the arch anatomy. A Judkins right 4 or internal mammary catheter or an angled steerable wire can be used. In a difficult anatomy,

Table 1
Commercially available equipment for transradial lower extremity interventions

Stent/Manufacturer	Shaft Length (cm)	Wire (in)	6-Fr Compatible Size (mm)	Length (mm)
Balloon				
Evercross	135	0.035	4–10	20–200
Mustang BSC	135	0.035	5–8	20–150
Sterling	150	0.035	2–7	20–150
Admiral Medtronic	130	0.035	4–10	20–200
Self-expanding stents				
Protégé (EV3)	150	0.035	5–14	20–120
IDEV	135	0.014	5–8	20–120
Complete (M)	130	0.035	5–10	20–120
Viabahn	120	0.018	5–6	50, 100, 150
Balloon-expandable stents				
Cobalt	135	0.035	5–10	20, 30, 40, 60
Visipro	135	0.035	5–8	17, 27, 37, 47
Express LD	150	0.018	6–8	17–57
ICAST (Atrium)	120	0.35	5–6	16, 22, 38

Device Purpose	Shaft Length (cm)	Wire (in)	6 Fr-Comp Diameter (mm)	Length (mm)
Atherectomy				
LASER	135	0.014	0.09–2.4	0.9, 1.7, 2
Flextom	137	0.018	3.5–6	10, 15, 40, 100
Angiosculpt	135	0.014	4–6	20, 40
CSI	150	0.014		
CTO				
True Path	165	0.018	NA	NA
Wild/KittyCat	150	0.018		
Frontrunner	140	0.014/0.035		
Outback	120	0.014		
Viance	150	0.014		
Enteer	150	0.014		
Distal protection				
SPIDER	320/190	0.014	4–7	NA
FILTER EZ	300	0.014	3.5–5.5	
NAV 3	325	0.014	5–6	

From Sanghvi K, Nachtigall J, Luft U. Transradial endovascular treatment of severe common femoral artery stenosis. J Invasive Cardiol 2013;25(11):616–9; with permission.

use a pigtail catheter and torque the catheter to have the pigtail face toward the descending aorta. Then use a 0.035″ wire to open the pigtail toward the descending aorta.

SUBCLAVIAN INTERVENTIONS
Indications and Prevalence
Subclavian interventions are most commonly performed to improve flow into the left internal mammary artery to allow for the use of the mammary artery for a bypass graft or to improve flow

into an artery already used for bypass grafting. Disease of the brachiocephalic arteries and subclavian artery is common in patients with PVD and the left subclavian ostia is most commonly affected. Other indications for intervention include syncope or light headiness owing to subclavian steal, arm claudication, or the need to improve forearm perfusion to allow for the creation of an arteriovenous fistula for dialysis. Prasad and colleagues[12] reported the prevalence of left subclavian stenosis to be 2.7% in patients undergoing preoperative coronary angiography. In patients with known PVD, the prevalence of subclavian stenosis is reported to be 19%.[13] Using a difference of 15 mm Hg blood pressure between arms for screening, Aboyans and colleagues[14] reported an 8.8% incidence of subclavian stenosis. As the population ages and the number of patients with coronary disease and peripheral disease increase, the need for subclavian interventions may rise to salvage prior left internal mammary grafts.

Endovascular subclavian intervention has become the mainstay of the treatment over surgical treatment. There are no randomized trials comparing balloon angioplasty, stenting, primary stenting, or provisional stenting, but stent placement currently remains a mainstay of treatment with a high initial success and good long-term success. A comprehensive review[15] of published series of patients treated with stents showed technical success achieved in 97%. Adverse events rates were 6% and most complications were minor and limited to vascular access difficulty and stent dislodgment. No strokes or death and 3% restenosis rate were reported.[15] In a small series[16] of 21 patients treated with subclavian interventions via femoral access, 2 of 21 patients had hematomas and 1 required treatment of an associated pseudoaneurysm.

With an increase in the number of radial procedures being performed for diagnostic and interventional coronary procedures owing to the decrease in access site and bleeding complications, it was natural to extend this access to subclavian interventions. Yu and colleagues[17] reported a case series of 14 patients undergoing subclavian intervention at a single center with a success rate of 93% and no access site complications.

Advantages of Radial Access for Subclavian Intervention

- The ipsilateral RA approach provides easy access and avoids the manipulation of catheters in the aortic arch, where the prevalence of calcified atherosclerotic plaques is high.
- Atherosclerotic disease of the subclavian artery commonly involves the ostial and proximal portions (Fig. 4). The radial approach provides better support to cross through a stenosis or chronic total occlusion and deliver balloons or stents. From the femoral approach, selective placement of the catheter or sheath is more challenging (Fig. 5, Videos 2 and 3; available online at http://www.interventional.theclinics.com/).
- Patients can be discharged home immediately after removing the hemostatic radial band.

Procedure

- Using the radial approach avoids access complications, allows early ambulation, and offers very stable guide support for subclavian interventions.
- At times, owing to the stenosis of the subclavian artery, the radial pulse may be difficult to palpate and ultrasound guidance maybe needed for obtaining ipsilateral radial artery access.

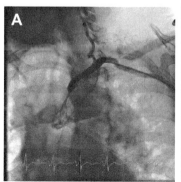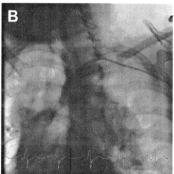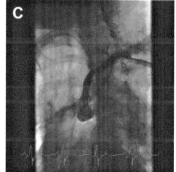

Fig. 4. (A) Initial control angiogram of the left subclavian shows severe ostial stenosis. (B) Stent placement in the subclavian using a multipurpose catheter. (C) Final result after treatment of the subclavian.

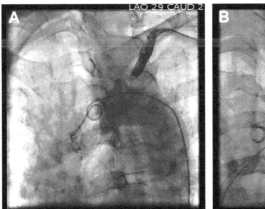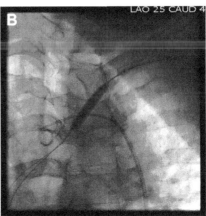

Fig. 5. (*A*) Left subclavian short segmental occlusion defined with simultaneous dual injection using a pigtail from the common femoral artery and multipurpose catheter from left radial. (*B*) Stent placement in left subclavian ostia guided by aorta angiography.

- Radial access is obtained in a standard fashion and, after insertion of a short sheath, a vasodilator cocktail is given followed by a diagnosis angiogram of using a 100-cm, 5-Fr, multipurpose catheter.
- After the anatomy of the lesion is established the short 5-Fr sheath is exchanged for at least a 65-cm, 6-Fr hydrophilic sheath, which is advanced to just distal to the lesion.
- The lesion is crossed with a guide wire and predilated with an undersized balloon. The balloon is removed and a 5-Fr pigtail catheter is advanced into the aortic arch, where an aortography is performed to help localize the disease in aortosubclavian ostium.
- For ostial lesions, the authors prefer to use balloon-expandable stents; if the lesion is not a true aorto-ostial disease and a variation in size of the proximal to distal artery is seen, a self-expanding stent can be used. With significant subclavian stenosis, a reversal of flow in the vertebral artery is most often present; therefore, protection devices are not used. At times, a contralateral radial or femoral access is used to advance a pigtail catheter to define the ostium of the subclavian artery (see **Fig. 5**, Videos 2 and 3; available online at http://www.interventional.theclinics.com/).

TRANSRADIAL CAROTID INTERVENTION
Indications and Guidelines
The advances in the carotid artery stenting (CAS) technology, techniques, and experience along with its less invasive nature have made CAS an attractive option for many patients. Numerous clinical trials have been performed to assess the safety and efficacy of the CAS, including those randomized 1 to 1 with carotid endarterectomy (CEA). Evidence for carotid stenting is plagued with heterogeneity in the study designs, operator experience, and embolic protection device use.[18–20] Nonetheless, major randomized trials such as SAPPHIRE,[21] CAPTURE,[22] and CREST[23] compared CAS and CEA for treating symptomatic and asymptomatic carotid artery stenosis patients and showed noninferiority of CAS. CAS is indicated (class I, level of evidence B)[24] as an alternative to CEA for symptomatic patients at average or low risk of complications associated with endovascular intervention and with 70% stenosis by noninvasive imaging or 50% stenosis by catheter angiography when the anticipated rate of periprocedure stroke or mortality is less than 6%. It is reasonable to choose CEA over CAS (class IIA, level of evidence B)[24] when revascularization is indicated in older patients, particularly when arterial pathoanatomy is unfavorable for endovascular intervention. Similarly it is reasonable to choose CAS over CEA (class IIA, level of evidence B)[24] when revascularization is indicated in patients with neck anatomy unfavorable for arterial surgery. Prophylactic CAS might be considered (class IIB, level of evidence B)[24] in highly selected patients with asymptomatic carotid stenosis (minimum 60% by angiography, 70% by validated Doppler ultrasonography), but its effectiveness compared with medical therapy alone in this situation is not well-established.

Advantages of Radial Access

Some of the anatomic variations of the aortic arch, common carotid artery, and/or presence of severe peripheral artery disease may make it difficult or impossible to use the default femoral access for CAS procedure. The well-understood safety related to the radial access and multiple feasibility studies[25–33] suggest that radial access could be an alternative strategy for carotid interventions, and may be a preferred approach in very experienced hands for treating right internal carotid artery disease, bovine left internal carotid disease, or in patients with severe PVD. Very high success rates (up to 92%) have been reported in these feasibility studies.[25–33] The use of the TR approach in patients with right internal carotid artery disease and bovine left internal carotid disease may reduce catheter-induced embolization from the traversing the aortic arch. Early ambulation and significantly reduced vascular access complications are the other advantages.

Procedure Tips and Tricks

- Operator should have extensive CAS experience and extensive experience using radial access for coronary and peripheral intervention procedures because all the feasibility studies had these 2 essential components.
- An arch aortogram is an important consideration.
- Considerations in catheter selection include:
  ○ Simmons 1, Simmons 2, or Tiger catheter are helpful cannulating the nonbovine left carotid artery (Videos 4.1 and 4.2; available online at http://www.interventional.theclinics.com/).
  ○ Judkin's right, internal mammary catheter, Amplantz right, or Simmons would work for the right carotid artery and bovine left carotid artery (see Video 4.4; available online at http://www.interventional.theclinics.com/)
  ○ A Tiger, Simmons 1 or 2 and Judkin's left curve may work with contralateral radial approach (see Video 4.3; Video 5; available online at http://www.interventional.theclinics.com/).[9]
  ○ Simmons 3 may be useful in extreme angles such as type III arch.
  ○ In difficult cases a 5- or 6-Fr guide catheter could be used for intermediary exchange of a 0.035″ stiff (Amplantz, Supra Core) wire and

telescopic technique to advance the sheath over the guide catheter can be a solution.

- Catheter Looping and Retrograde Engagement Technique (CLARET)[27] has a high success rate as an alternative strategy for TR CAS. The length of the catheter needed is a consideration in tall patients with a long arm span.

TRANSRADIAL RENAL AND SPLANCHNIC ARTERY CATHETERIZATION

Indication for Renal Artery Catheterization and Interventions

Although modern, multicenter, prospective registries demonstrated improvement of blood pressure control with renal artery revascularization with excellent safety,[34] recent randomized trials[35–37] have failed to establish a clear advantage in blood pressure control with renal artery stenting. These studies have been criticized for serious methodologic flaws in their design and execution of the studies with selection bias, lack of a core laboratory analysis, and enrolling patients where the significance of the lesion was unknown.[38] It seems that, in appropriately selected patients with hemodynamically significant renal artery stenosis, renal stenting improves blood pressure control, heart failure symptoms, and stabilizes chronic renal insufficiency.[37,39–41] Renal interventions have been shown to reduce the heart failure admission and/or episodes of flash pulmonary edema in selected patient.[37,39–41] Patients with accelerated or resistant hypertension (failure of_3 maximally tolerated medications including the use of a diuretic), global renal ischemia (bilateral renal artery stenosis or severe renal artery stenosis in a solitary functioning kidney), or hypertension with medication intolerance also generally benefit from renal artery stenting after a trial of optimal medical therapy; the patients excluded or not studied in the CORAL trial.

Indications for Splanchnic Artery Intervention

Acute intestinal ischemia because of the systemic thromboembolism or chronic intestinal ischemia, either because of the atherosclerotic superior mesenteric artery stenosis or compression of the celiac artery in arcuate ligament syndrome are the common indications for endovascular intervention. Chronic mesenteric ischemia occurs when 2 of the 3 major splanchnic arteries have severe stenosis. Female patients in their 50s and 60s are most commonly affected. Patients typically present with postprandial abdominal pain, sitophobia, and weight loss.

Advantages of Radial Approach for Renal and Splanchnic Interventions

Because of the high prevalence of atherosclerosis of the abdominal aorta abdominal aortography is recommended before selective renal catheterization to reduce the risk of renal artery injury and atheroembolization. A radiological study of renal artery origin reported a mean angle made by the right and the left renal artery with aorta is 73° and 65°, respectively (Fig. 6).[42] Similarly, the celiac and superior mesenteric artery origins form a caudally directed acute angle between 38° and 56° (see Fig. 6). The caudally directed openings of the renal and splanchnic arteries require a catheter with a steep curve (similar to renal double curve, hockey stick) from femoral approach, which still may not provide adequate support, and the catheter entry into the renal artery can be traumatic, particularly in difficult anatomy, because of the high prevalence of atheromatous disease. From the radial approach, the Judkins right or Multipurpose guide catheter allows relatively easy, atraumatic, coaxial, supportive engagement in renal and splanchnic vessels.[43]

Studies of renal stenting via a femoral approach have reported an access-related complication rate of up to 28%.[7] This may be expected, because high blood pressure is predictor of access site complications. Although brachial access offers the advantage of a craniocaudal approach, it too is associated with an high risk of access site complications. Several series using brachial access for coronary angiography reported complication rates as high as 7% to 11 %, including brachial artery thrombosis as the most commonly reported (1%–6%) serious complication.[44] Reductions in access-related complications, immediate ambulation, and early discharge associated with radial access can reduce cost and improved clinical outcomes.

Technical Tips for Performing the Procedure

- The left radial access is preferred because it reduces the need to traverse the aortic arch and allows for 10 cm more of working catheter length. A 110-cm-long guide catheter will reach the renal artery from left radial approach in most patients. Right radial access may be preferable to reduce operator radiation exposure. Very rarely, a longer catheter (>110 cm from left or >125 cm from right) may be required in patients with severe tortuosity of thoracic and abdominal aorta from the radial access.
- Tips to enter the descending aorta were described elsewhere in this article. The passage of the guide wire down the descending aorta has to be followed carefully to avoid injury to the branches of the aorta. A Judkins right 4 or Multipurpose catheter can be used to engage the renal arteries with a high success rate, preferably guided by aortography (Video 6; available online at http://www.interventional.theclinics.com/). The celiac artery and superior mesenteric artery can be engaged with a Multipurpose II or III catheter (Video 7; available online at http://www.interventional.theclinics.com/).
- Because of the supportive coaxial position of the guide catheter, a 0.014″ support

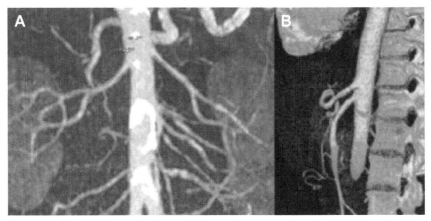

Fig. 6. Caudally directed angle of origin for the renal (A) superior mesenteric and celiac (B) arteries. (From Sanghvi K. Ten critical lessons for performing transradial catheterization. Endovascular Today 2014.)

wire is adequate for intervention in most cases (see Video 6; available online at http://www.interventional.theclinics.com/).

- Multiple commercially available stents can be used through a 6-Fr guide catheter or a 5-Fr sheath (Table 2). Depending on the guide length, a balloon, stent, or other device requires 120 or 135 cm of working shaft length.
- If use of a covered stent is desired, 1 of the 2 techniques can be used. A 6-Fr, 110-cm sheath can be telescoped over a 6-Fr guide catheter in to renal or splanchnic artery (Fig. 7) or previously described technique to use a 7-Fr guide catheter (see Fig. 1).

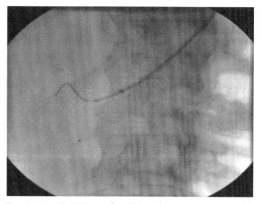

Fig. 7. A 6-Fr, 90-cm sheath is advanced over a multi-purpose guide catheter into the right renal artery.

LOWER EXTREMITY INTERVENTIONS
Aorta–Iliac Disease
Very often, iliac disease is associated with multi-level vascular disease and carries a much greater risk for cardiovascular events than small vessel PVD. Emerging data continue to challenge the current American Heart Association/American College of Cardiology guidelines recommending surgery for complex lesions.[45] The initial success rate as well as 1- and 5-year patency rates were not different while treating Trans-Atlantic Inter-Society Consensus (TASC) A or B versus TASC C or D aortoiliac lesions.[46]

Radial Approach
Flachskampf and colleagues[47] first reported on TR stenting of the iliac artery in 2005. The authors felt the radial approach would avoid damage to the disease femoral arteries, obviate the need to compress the femoral artery distal to a newly placed stent, and provide excellent support for delivery of balloons and stents as opposed to having to cross over from the opposite side. Sanghvi and colleagues[48] reported a retrospective review of 159 iliac and superficial femoral artery (SFA) interventions, of which 15 were performed via the radial approach. The access site was chosen at the operator's discretion for severe bilateral disease, absent femoral pulses, morbid obesity, or an inability to tolerate prolonged bed rest. Of the 15 patients, 14 had successful completion of the procedure; the 1 failure was owing to the need to treat a distal SFA lesion. The radial approach was safe with no access site complication and provided excellent support. Staniloae and associates[49] reported on a series of iliac interventions in 74 patients, 27 procedures were performed via the left RA. More patients (36%) in the transradial approach group had TASC C and D lesion compared with 19% for the transfemoral group. Success rates

| | | | | Sizes, mm (6-Fr | |
Stent	Manufacturer	Shaft Length (cm)	Wire (in)	Guide or 5-Fr Sheath Compatible)	Stent Lengths (mm)
Hippocampus	Invatec (Roncadelle, Italy)	145	0.014	4–7	10, 15, 20, 24
Palmaz-Genesis	Cordis (Fremont, CA)	142	0.014	4–6.5	12, 18
Herculink	Abbott Vascular (Santa Clara, CA)	135	0.014	4–7	12, 15, 18
Express SD	Boston Scientific (Marlborough, MA)	150	0.014	4–6	15, 18
Tsunami	Terumo (Somerset, NJ)	150	0.014	4–6	12, 18

Table 2
Commercially available renal stents with a 6-Fr guide catheter compatibility

From Sanghvi K, Coppola J, Patel T. Cranio-caudal (transradial) approach for renal artery intervention. J Interv Cardiol 2013;26(5):530–5; with permission.

were similar between the radial and femoral groups, although the femoral group had 7% minor access site complications compared with no access site complications for the radial group. Despite a slightly more complex mix, the procedure and fluoroscopy times and contrast were no different. With greater experience, there was an important 25-minute shortening of procedure times from the initial cases to the latest cases.

Femoral–Popliteal Disease

Claudication or critical limb ischemia caused by common femoral artery (CFA) disease is preferably treated by surgery because of the easy accessibility and favorable long-term outcomes of endarterectomy.[50] However, endovascular treatment of CFA disease with atherectomy, balloon angioplasty, and provisional stenting is also associated with a high success rate, low rate of in-hospital complications, and acceptable restenosis rate at medium-term follow-up.[51]

Radial Approach

CFA intervention is challenged by limited access choices in the presence of bilateral femoral artery disease. The limitation of CFA or SFA intervention from the radial approach is the availability of working length of the equipment and compatibility with a 6-Fr sheath in the United States. We have listed currently available equipment compatible with TR use in Table 1. Angioplasty balloon catheters of 150 cm are available and allow treatment of SFA lesions and are useful for treating in stent restenosis (Video 8; available online at http://www.interventional.theclinics.com/). The orbital atherectomy system is compatible with a 6-Fr sheath and has a workable length of 143 cm, which will reach the CFA and initial portion of the SFA in all but the tallest patients. For severe calcified disease in the CFA or proximal SFA, the orbital atherectomy could be used via TR approach successfully (Video 9; available online at http://www.interventional.theclinics.com/).[52] Trani and colleagues[53] described the use of a new 5-Fr compatible 180-cm-long self-expanding stent, the SuprFlex518, (Optimed, Ettlinger Germany).

Advantages of Radial Access for Lower Extremity Interventions

- The very few access-related complications are the most attractive reason for using radial access.

- Avoid difficult sheath placement when external iliac lesion is close to sheath insertion site when using ipsilateral approach.
- In the presence of severe tortuosity and heavy calcification of the iliac arteries, the usual crossover technique is very difficult. The geometry of a straight line from a sheath in the aorta or iliac artery to the target disease in the iliac or femoral artery provides very strong support (Video 10; available online at http://www.interventional.theclinics.com/). An example of solid support is seen in this case, where 0.035″ coils are deployed to treat internal iliac artery aneurysm via a left radial approach (Video 11; available online at http://www.interventional.theclinics.com/).
- Radial access eliminates the need of compression of the femoral artery after fresh stent placement in the ipsilateral iliac artery.
- Radial access allows immediate ambulation and same-day discharge after removing the hemostatic band 2 hours after the procedure, further reducing morbidity and the cost of the procedure.

Procedure

- Left radial access is preferred for lower extremity interventions because it eliminates the need to cross the aortic arch vessels and is a shorter distance to the descending aorta.
- Advance a 0.035″ J tip guide wire and a pigtail or multipurpose catheter to the descending aorta by using one of the tricks described earlier. Follow the passage of wire in aorta on fluoroscopy to avoid inadvertent passage in to branches of the thoracic or abdominal aorta.
- Abdominal aortography and lower extremity runoff angiography can be obtained by positioning the pigtail catheter appropriately to define aneurysms, collaterals, and the presence of ostial disease. A 125-cm, multipurpose catheter could be exchanged for selective iliac or CFA angiography. A 135- or 150-cm exchange catheter (listed in Table 1) can be used for selective angiography of SFA or popliteal when required.

- After defining the anatomy and crossing the lesion with a multipurpose catheter, a 300-cm support 0.035″ wire is secured beyond the lesion. A 5- or 6-Fr, 110-cm sheath is advanced into the target iliac artery or distal abdominal aorta. The sheath offers excellent support for the passage of wirers, balloons, and stents (Fig. 8).
- With self-expanding stents up to 14 mm diameter and balloon expandable stents up to 10 mm can be used through the 6-Fr sheath (see Table 1).
- The major limitation of this procedure is severe tortuosity of the left subclavian artery or descending aorta in which case the 110-cm sheath will not be long enough to reach the iliac artery. At times, placing a stiff guide wire in the long sheath can straighten the tortuosity and allow the sheath to reach the iliac artery.

- If bilateral iliac or external iliac disease is present, both sides can be treated in a consecutive fashion.
- If a kissing balloon procedure is needed, a 5-Fr catheter can be advanced via the right RA and exchange length wire placed in the contralateral iliac artery and the catheter removed a balloon can be passed over this wire without a sheath. Injections can be performed via the prior placed sheath.
- When facing a total obstruction, a 6-Fr sheath gives better support and allows for the use of reentry devices and, if needed, atherectomy devices (see Video 10).
- Before removal of the long sheath, additional conscious sedation or pain medication should be given. Spasm is very common with long, bulky sheaths. The sheath is removed with a slow, continuous, gentle pullback pressure. An additional dose of sublingual

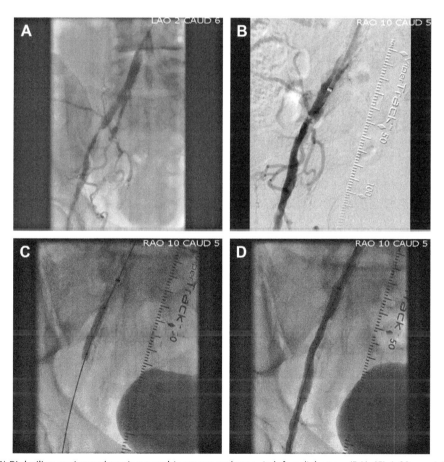

Fig. 8. (A) Right iliac angiography using a multipurpose catheter via left radial artery (RA). (B) A 90-cm, 6-Fr sheath is advanced into the right iliac artery. (C) Balloon angioplasty of the external iliac lesion. (D) Final angiography after self-expanding stent deployed in the right external iliac artery via the left RA.

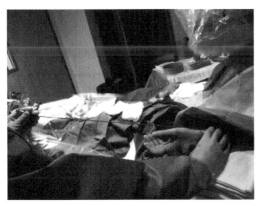

Fig. 9. A sheath measuring 90 cm is being removed with a slow, continuous pullback.

nitroglycerin helps. After pulling back the sheath into RA, aspirate 10 mL of blood forcefully and flush it with heparinized saline. An additional dose of exit vasodilator cocktail (nitroglycerin 200 µg and verapamil 2.5 mg) is recommended. A hemostatic band is applied and the rest of the sheath can be removed (Fig. 9).

SUMMARY

The use of the RA for peripheral procedures is a natural outgrowth of the increased utilization of radial access for coronary interventions. Although there are multiple case series or single-center experiences suggesting high success rate, feasibility, and reduced vascular access complications with TR endovascular interventions for the PVD, there are no randomized, controlled trials to date evaluating vascular access. The lack of concerted interest from the device industry also has challenged the expansion of TR use for endovascular interventions.

The advantages of access site safety, immediate ambulation, same-day discharge, cost savings, patient comfort, and quality of life improvement, as well as the suggested increase in the efficiency for some of the vascular bed are potential reasons to use radial access for peripheral procedures. With improving technology, techniques, experience, and training, radial access will likely continue to be adopted for procedures beyond the coronary bed.

SUPPLEMENTARY DATA

Supplementary data related to this article can be found online at http://dx.doi.org/10.1016/j.iccl.2015.01.003.

REFERENCES

1. Dehmer GJ, Weaver D, Roe MT, et al. A contemporary view of diagnostic cardiac catheterization and percutaneous coronary intervention in the United States: a report from the CathPCI Registry of the National Cardiovascular Data Registry, 2010 through June 2011. J Am Coll Cardiol 2012;60(20):2017–31.
2. Caputo RP, Tremmel JA, Patel T, et al. Transradial arterial access for coronary and peripheral procedures: executive summary by the transradial committee of the SCAI. Catheter Cardiovasc Interv 2011;78:823–39.
3. Hamon M, Pristipino C, Di Mario C, et al. Consensus document on the radial approach in percutaneous cardiovascular interventions: position paper by the European Association of Percutaneous Cardiovascular Interventions and Working Groups on Acute Cardiac Care and Thrombosis of the European Society of Cardiology. EuroIntervention 2013;8(11):1242–51.
4. Feldman DN, Swaminathan RV, Kaltenbach LA, et al. Adoption of radial access and comparison of outcomes to femoral access in percutaneous coronary intervention: an updated report from the national cardiovascular data registry (2007–2012). Circulation 2013;127:2295–306.
5. De Belder AJ, Smith RE, Wainwright RJ, et al. Transradial artery coronary angiography and intervention in patients with severe peripheral vascular disease. Clin Radiol 1997;52(2):115–8.
6. Judkins M, Gander M. Prevention of complications of coronary arteriography. Circulation 1974;49:599–602.
7. Samal AK, White CJ. Percutaneous management of access site complications. Catheter Cardiovasc Interv 2002;57:12–23.
8. Garcia S, McFalls EO, Goldman S, et al. Diagnostic coronary angiography in patients with peripheral arterial disease: a sub-study of the Coronary Artery Revascularization Prophylaxis Trial. J Interv Cardiol 2008;21:369–74.
9. Hildick-Smith DJ, Walsh JT, Lowe MD, et al. Coronary angiography in the presence of peripheral vascular disease: femoral or brachial/radial approach? Catheter Cardiovasc Interv 2000;49:32–7.
10. Hirsch AT, Criqui MH, Treat-Jacobson D, et al. Peripheral arterial disease detection, awareness, and treatment in primary care. JAMA 2001;286(11):1317–24.
11. Shammas NW. "Epidemiology, classification, and modifiable risk factors of peripheral arterial disease". Vasc Health Risk Manag 2007;3(2):229–34.
12. Prasad A, Prasad A, Varghese I, et al. Prevalence and treatment of proximal left subclavian artery stenosis in patients referred for coronary artery bypass surgery. Int J Cardiol 2009;133:109–11.

13. Gutierrez GR, Mahrer P, Aharonian V, et al. Prevalence of subclavian artery stenosis in patients with peripheral vascular disease. Angiology 2001;52:189–94.

14. Aboyans V, Criqui MH, Mc Dermott MM, et al. The vital prognosis of subclavian stenosis. J Am Coll Cardiol 2007;49:1540–5.

15. Hadjipetrou P, Cox S, Piemonte T, et al. Percutaneous revascularization of atherosclerotic obstruction of aortic arch vessels. J Am Coll Cardiol 1999;33:1238–45.

16. Angle JF, Matsumoto A, McGraw JK, et al. Percutaneous angioplasty and stenting of the left subclavian artery stenosis in patients with left internal mammary-coronary by-pass grafts: clinical experience and long term follow up. Vasc Endovascular Surg 2003;37:89–97.

17. Yu J, Korabathina R, Coppola J, et al. Transradial approach to subclavian artery stenting. J Invasive Cardiol 2010;22:204–6.

18. Mas JL, Chatellier G, Beyssen B, et al. Endarterectomy versus stenting in patients with symptomatic severe carotid stenosis. N Engl J Med 2006;355:1660–71.

19. Ederle J, Dobson J, Featherstone RL, et al. Carotid artery stenting compared with endarterectomy in patients with symptomatic carotid stenosis (internal carotid stenting study): an interim analysis of a randomized controlled trial. Lancet 2010;375:985–97.

20. Ringleb PA, Allenberg J, Bruckmann H, et al. 30 day results from the SPACE trial of stent-protected angioplasty versus carotid endarterectomy in symptomatic patients: a randomized non-inferiority trial. Lancet 2006;368:1239–47.

21. Yadav JS, Wholey MH, Kuntz RE, et al. Protected carotid-artery stenting versus endarterectomy in high-risk patients. N Engl J Med 2004;351:1493–501.

22. Gray WA, Rosenfield KA, Jaff MR, et al. Influence of site and operator characteristics on carotid artery stent outcome analysis of the capture 2 clinical study. JACC Cardiovasc Interv 2011;4:235–46.

23. Brott TG, Hobson RW 2nd, Howard G, et al. Stenting versus endarterectomy for treatment of carotid-artery stenosis (CREST). N Engl J Med 2010;363:11–23.

24. Brott TG, Halperin JL, Abbara S, et al. 2011 ASA/ACCF/AHA/AANN/AANS/ACR/ASNR/CNS/SAIP/SCAI/SIR/SNIS/SVM/SVS guideline on the management of patients with extracranial carotid and vertebral artery disease: executive summary. Catheter Cardiovasc Interv 2013;81:E75–123.

25. Folmar J, Sachar R, Mann T. Transradial approach for carotid artery stenting: a feasibility study. Catheter Cardiovasc Interv 2007;69:355–61.

26. Patel T, Shah S, Ranian A, et al. Contralateral transradial approach for carotid artery stenting: a feasibility study. Catheter Cardiovasc Interv 2009;75:268–75.

27. Fang H, Chung S, Sun C, et al. Transradial and transbrachial arterial approach for simultaneous carotid angiographic examination and stenting using catheter looping and retrograde engagement technique. Ann Vasc Surg 2010;24:670–9.

28. Mendiz OA, Sampaolesi AH, Londero HF, et al. Initial experience with transradial access for carotid stenting. Vasc Endovascular Surg 2011;45:499–503.

29. Pinter L, Cagiannos C, Ruzsa Z, et al. Report on initial experience with transradial access for carotid artery stenting. J Vasc Surg 2007;45:1136–41.

30. Bakoyiannis C, Economopoulos KP, Georgopoulos S, et al. Transradial access for carotid artery stenting: a single center experience. Int Angiol 2010;29:41–6.

31. Coroleu SF, Burzotta F, Fernández-Gómez C, et al. Feasibility of complex coronary and peripheral interventions by trans-radial approach using large sheathes. Catheter Cardiovasc Interv 2012;79:597–600.

32. Shaw JA, Gravereaux EC, Eisenhauer AC. Carotid stenting in the bovine arch. Catheter Cardiovasc Interv 2003;60:566–9.

33. Etxegoien N, Rhyne D, Kedev S, et al. The transradial approach for carotid artery stenting. Catheter Cardiovasc Interv 2012;80:1081–7.

34. Jaff MR, Bates M, Sullivan T, et al. Significant reduction in systolic blood pressure following renal artery stenting in patients with uncontrolled hypertension: results from the HERCULES trial. Catheter Cardiovasc Interv 2012;80:343–50.

35. Bax L, Woittiez AJ, Kouwenberg HJ, et al. Stent placement in patients with atherosclerotic renal artery stenosis and impaired renal function: a randomized trial. Ann Intern Med 2009;150:840–1.

36. Wheatley K, Ives N, Gray R, et al. Revascularization versus medical therapy for renal-artery stenosis. N Engl J Med 2009;361:1953–62.

37. Van Jaarsveld BC, Krijnen P, Pieterman H, et al. The effect of balloon angioplasty on hypertension in atherosclerotic renal-artery stenosis. Dutch Renal Artery Stenosis Intervention Cooperative Study Group. N Engl J Med 2000;342:1007–14.

38. Weinberg M, Olin J. Stenting for atherosclerotic renal artery stenosis: one poorly designed trial after another. Cleve Clin J Med 2010;77(3):164–71.

39. Kane G, Xu N, Roubicek T, et al. Renal artery revascularization improves heart failure control in patients with atherosclerotic renal artery stenosis. Nephrol Dial Transplant 2010;25:813–9.

40. Bloch M, Trost D, Pickering TG, et al. Prevention of recurrent pulmonary edema in patients with bilateral renovascular disease through renal artery stent placement. Am J Hypertens 1999;12:1–7.

41. Subramanian R, Silva JA, White CJ, et al. Stenting of renal artery stenosis preserves renal function in both diabetic and nondiabetic patients with

chronic renal insufficiency. J Am Coll Cardiol 2003; 41(6s1):75.

42. Garcier JM, De Fraissinette B, Filaire M, et al. Origin and initial course of the renal arteries: a radiologic study. Surg Radiol Anat 2001;23:51–5.

43. Sanghvi K, Coppola J, Patel T. Cranio-caudal (transradial) approach for renal artery intervention. J Interv Cardiol 2013;26(5):530–5.

44. Armstrong PJ, Han DC, Baxter JA, et al. Complication rates of percutaneous brachial artery access in peripheral vascular angiography. Ann Vasc Surg 2003;17(1):107–10.

45. Hirsch AT, Haskal ZJ, Hertzer NR, et al. ACC/AHA 2005 guidelines for the management of patients with peripheral arterial disease (lower extremity, renal, mesenteric and abdominal aortic. J Am Coll Cardiol 2006;47:1239–312.

46. Ichihashi S, Higashiura W, Itoh H, et al. Long-term outcomes for systematic primary stent placement in complex iliac artery occlusive disease classified according to the Trans-Atlantic Inter-Society Consensus (TASC II). J Vasc Surg 2011;53:992–9.

47. Flachskampf FA, Wolf T, Daniel WG, et al. Transradial stenting of the iliac artery: a case report. Catheter Cardiovasc Interv 2005;65:193–5.

48. Sanghvi K, Kurian D, Coppola J. Transradial intervention of iliac and superficial femoral artery disease is feasible. J Interv Cardiol 2008;21:385–7.

49. Staniloae C, Korabathina R, Yu J, et al. Safety and efficacy of transradial aortoiliac interventions. Catheter Cardiovasc Interv 2010;75:659–62.

50. Mukherjee D, Inahara T. Endarterectomy as the procedure of choice for atherosclerotic occlusive lesions of the common femoral artery. Am J Surg 1989;157:498–500.

51. Bonvini RF, Rastan A, Zeller T, et al. Endovascular treatment of common femoral artery disease: medium-term outcomes of 360 consecutive procedures. J Am Coll Cardiol 2011;58(8):792–8.

52. Sanghvi K, Nachtigall J, Luft U. Transradial endovascular treatment of severe common femoral artery stenosis. J Invasive Cardiol 2013;25(11):616–9.

53. Trani C, Tommasino A, Burzotta F. Pushing the limits forward: transradial superficial femoral artery stenting. Catheter Cardiovasc Interv 2010;76:1065–71.

Complications of Transradial Cardiac Catheterization and Management

Vinay Arora, MD[a,b], Meet Patel, MD[a,b],
Adhir R. Shroff, MD, MPH[a,b],*

KEYWORDS

- Transradial coronary angiography • Radial artery • Vascular access complications

---

KEY POINTS

- The transradial approach has become increasingly popular owing to decreased access site complications and length of hospital stay, and increased patient satisfaction.
- Complications are unique; common complications include radial artery occlusion and radial artery spasm.
- Less common complications include forearm hematoma and compartment syndrome, radial artery perforation, arteriovenous fistula formation, nerve damage, granuloma formation, and catheter entrapment.
- Recognition of these complications as well as preventive measures and management options are crucial to achieve procedural success.

INTRODUCTION

Historically the transfemoral approach for coronary angiography and percutaneous intervention has been the preferred method worldwide. Coronary angiography via a transradial approach was first described in 1989,[1] with the first successful transradial percutaneous coronary intervention taking place in 1993.[2] Multiple recent studies have shown reduced vascular access and bleeding complications, decreased hospital stays with resultant decreased health care costs, and increased patient satisfaction when comparing the transradial approach with the conventional transfemoral method.[3–5] Safety and effectiveness of the transradial approach have also been demonstrated in patients with acute coronary syndromes.[6] As such, it is not

surprising that the proportion of transradial percutaneous coronary intervention in the United States has increased from 1.2% in 2007 to 16.1% in 2012.[7] As this method continues to gain popularity, however, it is important to be cognizant of the potential complications of transradial procedures. In this article, we discuss the common and less common complications (Box 1) of transradial procedures, as well as strategies for prevention and management options.

RADIAL ARTERY OCCLUSION

Radial artery occlusion (RAO) is a well-recognized complication of transradial catheterization with variable reported incidence rates of anywhere from 1% to 38%.[8–10] Endothelial injury from sheath insertion and cessation of radial

---

The authors have nothing to disclose.
[a] Section of Cardiology, University of Illinois Hospital & Health Sciences System, 840 South Wood Street, MC 715, Chicago, IL 60612, USA; [b] Section of Cardiology, Jesse Brown VA Medical Center, 820 South Damen Avenue, Chicago, IL 60612, USA
* Corresponding author. 840 South Wood Street, MC 715, Chicago, IL 60612.
E-mail address: arshroff@uic.edu

artery flow create an environment conducive to thrombosis, which is thought to be the underlying process responsible for RAO.[11] RAO typically occurs early in the postprocedure setting, with many patients having spontaneous recanalization within 1 to 3 months.[12,13] RAO is often silent clinically, given the dual blood supply to the hand from the radial and ulnar arteries; however, case reports do exist of critical hand ischemia resulting from transradial procedures (Fig. 1).[14,15] The incidence of symptomatic

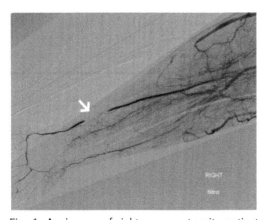

Fig. 1. Angiogram of right upper extremity patient with symptoms of hand ischemia revealing radial artery occlusion and small ulnar artery with diffuse spasm. Angiogram after intraarterial nitroglycerin administration showed radial artery occlusion (*arrow*) and a small ulnar artery with diffuse spasm. The patient had prolonged pain and ischemia of the fifth digit of her right hand. (*From* Kanei Y, Kwan T, Nakra NC, et al. Transradial cardiac catheterization: a review of access site complications. Catheter Cardiovasc Interv 2011;78:842; with permission.)

RAO requiring medical attention has been reported as 2% in the RIVAL study.[6]

Clinical implications of RAO include inability to utilize the radial artery in future catheterizations or as a bypass conduit. RAO also increases the theoretic risk of hand ischemia if the ipsilateral ulnar artery is utilized for subsequent vascular access. Several studies have identified independent predictors of RAO which include sheath size and sheath to artery ratio, postprocedure compression time, presence of anterograde flow during hemostasis, and use of systemic anticoagulation.

Sheath Size

The relationship between radial artery and sheath size as a predictor of RAO has been well-studied in the medical literature. The outer diameter of 5 French (Fr), 6-, 7-, and 8-Fr sheaths measure 2.28, 2.52, 2.85, and 3.22 mm, respectively. Saito and colleagues[16] used ultrasonography to evaluate radial artery size in comparison with sheath size in 250 Japanese patients undergoing transradial percutaneous coronary intervention. A significant difference was noted in severe flow reduction with a sheath-to-artery ratio of greater than 1 versus less than 1 (13% vs 4%; $P = .01$). Interestingly, 6-Fr sheaths were used in all patients successfully, even though only 86% of males and 73% of females in the study had a radial artery diameter larger than the external diameter of the sheath, demonstrating the artery's ability to stretch.

Uhlemann and colleagues[10] performed duplex ultrasonography before discharge in 455 patients who underwent transradial catheterization with either a 5- or 6-Fr sheath without initial evaluation of radial artery size. RAO was noted in 13.7% of patient with 5-Fr sheaths versus 30.5% in those with 6-Fr sheaths ($P<.001$). Another recent study comparing 4- with 6-Fr sheaths in transradial catheterization showed a reduction in RAO, however, did not attain significance.[17] Smaller sheath size has been shown to reduce the risk of RAO with comparable procedural success rates with those utilizing larger sheath sizes.[17,18]

Method of Hemostasis

Prolonged occlusion of the radial artery, particularly in the postprocedural setting while establishing hemostasis, has been shown to increase the risk of RAO. A decrease in the rate of RAO has been well-described with reduced hemostasis times as well as with maintained patency of the radial artery during hemostasis. Pancholy and colleagues[19] prospectively randomized 436 patients undergoing transradial catheterization into 2 groups based on method of hemostasis. Group I underwent conventional pressure application whereas group II underwent patent hemostasis, where radial artery patency was confirmed during pressure application. They found a significant difference in the rate of RAO between the conventional pressure group and the patent hemostasis group at both 24 hours and 30 days after the procedure (12% vs 5% [P<.05] and 7% vs 1.8% [P<.05], respectively). Approximately 43% of patients in group I had absence of forward flow during compression confirmed by the Barbeau test.[20] Of the patients in the conventional group who maintained patency during compression, 99.2% maintained radial patency at 30 days. There was no difference in the rate of bleeding complications, defined as blood loss leading to hemodynamic instability, transfusion, or death.

Having confirmed a reduction in RAO rates by patent hemostasis, the authors studied the effect of duration of hemostatic compression on RAO.[21] The rate of RAO was significantly less in a group of patients receiving 2 hours of hemostatic compression in comparison with a group receiving 6 hours (5.5% vs 12% [P = .025] and 3.5% vs 8.5% [P = .035], respectively). The only significant predictor of RAO at 30 days was absence of radial artery patency at the time of hemostatic compression.

Patent hemostasis has become the standard of care for postprocedural hemostasis and a variety of compressive wristbands now exist to ease the role of the operator in postprocedural hemostasis. Algorithms are in place for gradual deflation of these devices after compression time has completed. Compression times have also decreased and shorter durations of compression are now the norm.

Systemic Anticoagulation

Anticoagulation with heparin during diagnostic transradial catheterization was first shown to reduce RAO by Spaulding and colleagues[22] in a nonrandomized study in which patients received no heparin, 2000 to 3000 IU of heparin, or 5000 IU of heparin. Seventy-one percent of patients in the no heparin group, 24% in the low-dose heparin group, and 4.3% in the 5000 IU dose group were found to have RAO (P<.05). Approximately 75.8% of transradial operators worldwide have reported using 2000 to 5000 IU of heparin routinely in transradial cases.[23]

Although the conventional route of heparin administration has been intravenously, the intra-arterial approach is gaining popularity. A study comparing intravenous versus intra-arterial heparin showed no difference in RAO rates; however, patient discomfort associated with a burning sensation was more common with intra-arterial heparin.[24]

The role of alternate anticoagulants has also been evaluated in various studies. Both bivalirudin[25] and low-molecular-weight heparin[26] are also effective. In a recent case-control study, Pancholy and colleagues[27] compared RAO rates in patients on chronic warfarin therapy with therapeutic International Normalized Ratio values versus those not on chronic anticoagulation who received procedural unfractionated heparin during diagnostic transradial coronary angiography. They found a significantly lower rate of early and late RAO in the heparin group.

Treatment

RAO is often clinically silent owing to the dual blood supply to the hand and is thus underdiagnosed. In a study assessing RAO 3 to 4 hours after hemostatic compression, 1 hour of ipsilateral ulnar artery compression showed a reduction in the rate of RAO from 5.9% to 4.1% in patients who had received 2000 IU heparin and 2.9% to 0.8% in those who had received 5000 IU heparin.[28] In another study of patients with symptomatic RAO 1 day after transradial catheterization, treatment with low-molecular-weight heparin in symptomatic patients showed a significantly higher rate of partial or complete arterial recanalization at 4 weeks compared with no therapeutic anticoagulation in asymptomatic patients.[9] Conservative management with observation alone is common; however, in symptomatic patients or in those with further radial procedures planned, recanalization may be warranted. Revascularization techniques have been described with mixed outcomes.[29–31]

RADIAL ARTERY SPASM

Radial artery spasm (RAS) is another well-recognized complication of transradial catheterization procedures. The radial artery is composed mainly of smooth muscle cells arranged in concentric layers with a high density of alpha-1 receptors, which makes this vessel particularly prone to spasm.[32] Although RAS rarely results in serious complications, RAS decreases procedural success owing to difficulty obtaining radial access and increases difficulty of sheath removal upon case completion.

The incidence of RAS varies greatly in the current literature given the wide range of criteria used to define the phenomenon. Several studies have identified independent predictors of RAS including younger age, female gender, small radial artery size, anomalous radial artery anatomy, more than 3 catheter changes, and moderate to severe pain during cannulation.[33,34] Strategies to prevent occurrence of RAS include administration of intra-arterial vasodilators, utilization of hydrophilic-coated sheaths, and adequate operator training and experience with the transradial approach.

Vasodilator Therapy

Kiemeneij and colleagues[35] prospectively studied 100 patients undergoing transradial catheterization; one-half received intra-arterial verapamil and nitroglycerin and one-half received no vasodilator therapy. The investigators observed a reduction in maximal pullback force as well as patient pain during sheath removal in the group that received vasodilator therapy versus the group that did not (reported pain 14% vs 34% [$P = .019$], respectively).

In the SPASM 1 and 2 trials, RAS occurred in 22.2% of patients not receiving any vasodilator therapy before percutaneous coronary intervention.[36] A combination of molsidomine 1 mg and verapamil 2.5 mg was shown to reduce significantly the incidence of RAS (4.9%) compared with molsidomine or verapamil alone (13.3% vs 8.3%, respectively). No difference was noted between verapamil 2.5 versus 5 mg. SPASM 3 compared verapamil, diltiazem, and isosorbide dinitrate. The investigators showed a significant reduction in RAS by verapamil and isosorbitdinitrate compared with diltiazem.[37]

Vasodilator cocktails vary from practice to practice, with many high-volume transradial operators using no cocktail, which speaks to the role of operator experience in RAS. Of the various cocktails in practice, however, calcium channel blockers and nitrates have been shown most consistently to reduce the rate of RAS.

Sheath Selection

Sheaths with a hydrophilic coating are designed to decrease friction between the sheath and vessel walls, allowing for easier insertion and removal. In a randomized trial, Rathore and colleagues[38] investigated the effect of hydrophilic sheath coating as well as sheath length on the incidence of RAS. In this study, hydrophilic coated and uncoated sheaths of 13 and 23 cm in length were used. RAS, defined as moderate to severe discomfort on sheath withdrawal, was noted in 19% of patients with hydrophilic sheaths versus 39.9% of patients with uncoated

sheaths ($P<.001$). There was no difference in the rate of RAS between the 2 sheath lengths. Interestingly, a high incidence of local inflammatory reaction was seen in patients who received the hydrophilic sheath. Thought to be secondary to a local allergic reaction to residual hydrophilic polymer at the access site, there are no known long-term sequelae and patients are typically managed conservatively with analgesics and antibiotics.

Treatment

Prevention of RAS with the use of vasodilator cocktails and hydrophilic sheaths is key, although it is not always effective. Treatment strategies for sheath removal and resolution of RAS include repeat administration of intra-arterial vasodilator, additional sedation/analgesia, reinsertion of the introducer and guidewire, and often times merely operator patience. Case reports exist of alternative methods, including flow-mediated vasodilation, in which a blood pressure cuff is applied to the upper arm with a systolic pressure of 40 mm Hg above patient's systolic blood pressure for 5 minutes followed by release of cuff with gentle traction applied to the sheath.[39] In refractory cases, axillary nerve blocks or general anesthesia may be required.[40] Excessive force should never be applied, because this can lead to traumatic eversion endarterectomy.[41]

LESS COMMON COMPLICATIONS

Although RAO and RAS are the most recognized and described complications of transradial catheterization, other access site complications can occur, including forearm hematoma and compartment syndrome, radial artery perforation, arteriovenous fistula formation, nerve damage, granuloma formation, and catheter entrapment.

FOREARM HEMATOMA AND COMPARTMENT SYNDROME

The radial artery is a fairly superficial structure and thus has limited surrounding space to contain bleeding. Transradial access site bleeding, similar to femoral access site bleeding, is associated with long-term major adverse cardiac events.[42] If not controlled, bleeding can progress rapidly to hematoma formation. Female sex, sheath size, and procedure duration are factors associated with hematoma formation.[43,44]

The progression from hematoma to forearm compartment syndrome is very rare. In 1 case series, this progression occurred in less than 0.5% of cases.[43] There are 4 compartments in the forearm: dorsal, superficial volar, deep volar, and the mobile wad, each separated by tense fascia. As bleeding occurs in any of these compartments, pressure within the compartment increases, causing tissue edema and eventually ischemia and nerve damage.[45] Symptoms of compartment syndrome include forearm swelling and acute forearm pain. A high level of clinical suspicion is crucial to make a timely diagnosis because an unrecognized compartment syndrome can have devastating consequences. Compartment pressures can be measured to confirm the diagnosis, with a compartment pressure of greater than 30 mm Hg being consistent with compartment syndrome.

Prevention of compartment syndrome includes adequate vasodilator therapy before sheath removal, prompt recognition and treatment of hematomas, and continued monitoring of the patient for any worsening swelling or pain. Management is often conservative; however, surgical fasciotomy is required occasionally. The Early Discharge After Transradial Stenting of Coronary Arteries (EASY) trial[46] proposed a classification and treatment system for postprocedural hematoma (Fig. 2).

RADIAL ARTERY PERFORATION

Radial artery perforation is another rare complication seen with the transradial approach. Calvino Santos and colleagues[47] reported the incidence to be 1%, whereas in another large case series the incidence was closer to 0.1%.[48] Perforation occurs more often in elderly, short-statured women as well as in patients with tortuous and atherosclerotic arteries. Anatomic variations such as radial loops, a high radial–ulnar bifurcation, and a short ascending aorta also increase the risk of perforation.[49]

Various approaches can be used in the management of radial artery perforation. Calvino-Santos and associates[47] described a method of

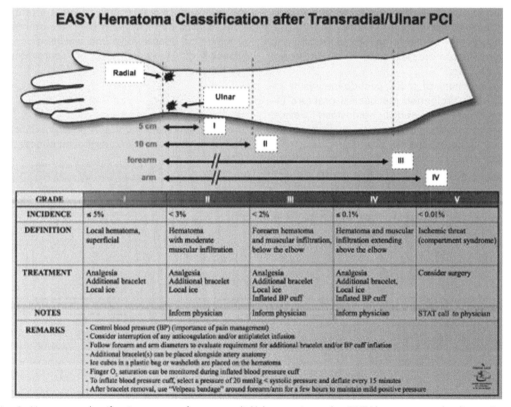

Fig. 2. Hematoma classification system after transradial/ulnar angiography. EASY hematoma scale: diagnosis and management (posters available upon request). [Color figure can be viewed in the online issue, which is available at: www.interscience.wiley.com]. (*From* Bertrand OF. Acute forearm muscle swelling post transradial catheterization and compartment syndrome: prevention is better than treatment! Catheter Cardiovasc Interv 2010;75:367; with permission.)

effectively sealing the perforation with a longer sheath, allowing for completion of the procedure via the radial artery. Angiography performed after the procedure showed no extravasation of contrast (Fig. 3). Furthermore, no major vascular complications developed during follow-up. In another approach, the guide catheter is used to seal the perforation allowing for procedure completion without sheath exchange.[50] A third approach using a balloon inflated for 5 minutes at the site of perforation has been shown to seal the perforation effectively.[51] Use of a coronary polytetrafluoroethylene-covered stent graft to reconstruct the perforated vessel has also been described.[52]

PSEUDOANEURYSM

The incidence of radial artery pseudoaneurysm has been shown to be less than 0.1% in a large case series.[48] Pseudoaneurysms usually present as a pulsatile mass with or without localized swelling and pain in the wrist, antecubital fossa, or forearm (Fig. 4). Diagnosis is made using Doppler ultrasonography or angiography. Although there have been no systematic studies analyzing the risk factors for radial artery pseudoaneurysms, systemic anticoagulation and inadequate compression have been suggested as risk factors.[53]

Management of radial pseudoaneurysms includes firm prolonged mechanical pressure (4–6 hours) with a radial hemostasis device, ultrasound-guided compression, thrombin injection, or surgical repair.[53–55] In the RIVAL trial,[6] pseudoaneurysms that required ultrasound compression, thrombin injection, or surgical repair occurred in 0.2% of transradial access patients versus 0.7% of transfemoral patients (P = .006). Early treatment can help to minimize complications, which may include tissue ischemia.

ARTERIOVENOUS FISTULA

Arteriovenous fistula formation in transradial procedures is an extremely rare complication given the superficial course of the vessel and the surrounding small caliber veins. While obtaining radial access, the initial puncture may deviate through a venous tributary and can lead to arteriovenous communication. These communications typically seal spontaneously; however, if they remain patent an arteriovenous fistula can form. Pain and swelling at the site can be seen with a palpable thrill. When this occurs, surgical repair is the usual approach, as seen in many case reports.[56–58] Surgical options vary depending on the size and location of the arteriovenous fistula. These options include partial resection, ligation, excision, and repair. Given the relatively benign course of most arteriovenous fistulas, there has also been a case report arguing for conservative management in the absence of increasing size or neurovascular insufficiency.[59]

NERVE DAMAGE

There are few major nerves in close proximity to the radial artery; however, digital numbness may

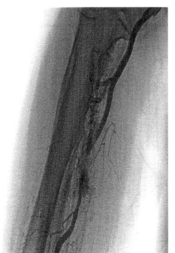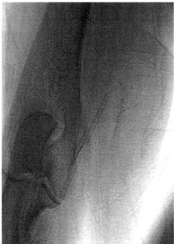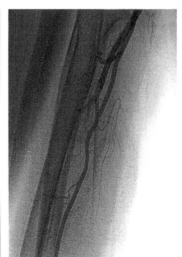

Fig. 3. Iatrogenic radial artery perforation (*left*) with long sheath insertion (*middle*) and subsequent resolution with no extravasation of contrast (*right*). Insertion of a long arterial sheath up to the brachial artery. (*From* Calvino-Santos RA, Vázquez-Rodríguez JM, Salgado-Fernández J, et al. Management of iatrogenic radial artery perforation. Catheter Cardiovasc Interv 2004;61:75, 76; with permission.)

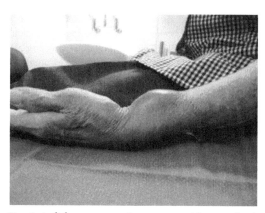

Fig. 4. Left forearm pseudoaneurysm with area of pulsatile swelling at radial access site. (*From* Collins N, Wainstein R, Ward M, et al. Pseudoaneurysm after transradial cardiac catheterization: case series and review of the literature. Catheter Cardiovasc Interv 2012;80:284; with permission.)

occur if the median or radial nerves are injured during repeated punctures. Complex regional pain syndrome of the hand is a more serious, yet still rare, complication after transradial catheterization. The exact incidence has not been studied, but case reports exist in the literature.[60–62] Management is usually conservative with the occasional need for sympathetic blockade.

GRANULOMA FORMATION

Several case studies have shown an association between hydrophilic sheaths and sterile granulomatous reactions at the access site. Histologic evaluations of these granulomas show foreign material underneath the skin, which is most likely owing to the sheath coating.[63,64] Typically occurring 2 to 3 weeks after the procedure, granulomas are self-limiting and are managed conservatively as long as patients do not develop signs or symptoms of infection.[65]

CATHETER ENTRAPMENT

Excessive catheter manipulation and tortuous vascular anatomy can lead to catheter kinking and subsequent catheter entrapment. Operator experience and early identification of catheter kinking are crucial in the avoidance of catheter entrapment. In such cases, gentle traction allows typically for straightening of the catheter. Additional support from a guidewire can also be useful. Percutaneous techniques have also been described in the event of unsuccessful conservative management. Specifically,

withdrawal of the catheter into the brachial artery can allow for fixation of the catheter either manually or with the assistance of a sphygmomanometer cuff. With the catheter fixed in place, it can be rotated proximally allowing for reduction of the knot.[66,67] Furthermore, a secondary access site may be used to introduce a snare to fix the tip of the catheter for it to be unwound.

SUMMARY

Transradial coronary angiography and percutaneous intervention is continuing to gain momentum in the United States owing to decreased bleeding and access site complications, reduced hospital stays and health care costs, and increased patient satisfaction compared with the conventional transfemoral approach. However, the transradial approach brings its own challenges and complications to the table. Recognition of these challenges as well as knowledge of strategies for prevention and management options is of the utmost importance for the modern-day clinician to deliver the highest level of patient care possible.

REFERENCES

1. Campeau L. Percutaneous radial artery approach for coronary angiography. Cathet Cardiovasc Diagn 1989;16(1):3–7.
2. Kiemeneij F, Laarman GJ. Percutaneous transradial artery approach for coronary stent implantation. Cathet Cardiovasc Diagn 1993;30(2):173–8.
3. Burzotta F, Trani C, Mazzari MA, et al. Vascular complications and access crossover in 10,676 transradial percutaneous coronary procedures. Am Heart J 2012;163(2):230–8.
4. Jolly SS, Amlani S, Hamon M, et al. Radial versus femoral access for coronary angiography or intervention and the impact on major bleeding and ischemic events: a systematic review and meta-analysis of randomized trials. Am Heart J 2009; 157(1):132–40.
5. Eichhofer J, Horlick E, Ivanov J, et al. Decreased complication rates using the transradial compared to the transfemoral approach in percutaneous coronary intervention in the era of routine stenting and glycoprotein platelet IIb/IIIa inhibitor use: a large single-center experience. Am Heart J 2008;156(5): 864–70.
6. Jolly SS, Yusuf S, Cairns J, et al. Radial versus femoral access for coronary angiography and intervention in patients with acute coronary syndromes

(RIVAL): a randomised, parallel group, multicentre trial. Lancet 2011;377(9775):1409–20.

7. Feldman DN, Swaminathan RV, Kaltenbach LA, et al. Adoption of radial access and comparison of outcomes to femoral access in percutaneous coronary intervention: an updated report from the national cardiovascular data registry (2007-2012). Circulation 2013;127(23):2295–306.

8. Tuncez A, Kaya Z, Aras D, et al. Incidence and predictors of radial artery occlusion associated transradial catheterization. Int J Med Sci 2013; 10(12):1715–9.

9. Zankl AR, Andrassy M, Volz C, et al. Radial artery thrombosis following transradial coronary angiography: incidence and rationale for treatment of symptomatic patients with low-molecular-weight heparins. Clin Res Cardiol 2010;99(12):841–7.

10. Uhlemann M, Möbius-Winkler S, Mende M, et al. The Leipzig prospective vascular ultrasound registry in radial artery catheterization: impact of sheath size on vascular complications. JACC Cardiovasc Interv 2012;5(1):36–43.

11. Kotowycz MA, Dzavik V. Radial artery patency after transradial catheterization. Circ Cardiovasc Interv 2012;5(1):127–33.

12. Stella PR, Kiemeneij F, Laarman GJ, et al. Incidence and outcome of radial artery occlusion following transradial artery coronary angioplasty. Cathet Cardiovasc Diagn 1997;40(2):156–8.

13. Nagai S, Abe S, Sato T, et al. Ultrasonic assessment of vascular complications in coronary angiography and angioplasty after transradial approach. Am J Cardiol 1999;83(2):180–6.

14. Taglieri N, Galie N, Marzocchi A. Acute hand ischemia after radial intervention in patient with CREST-associated pulmonary hypertension: successful treatment with manual thromboaspiration. J Invasive Cardiol 2013;25(2):89–91.

15. Kanei Y, Kwan T, Nakra NC, et al. Transradial cardiac catheterization: a review of access site complications. Catheter Cardiovasc Interv 2011;78(6): 840–6.

16. Saito S, Ikei H, Hosokawa G, et al. Influence of the ratio between radial artery inner diameter and sheath outer diameter on radial artery flow after transradial coronary intervention. Catheter Cardiovasc Interv 1999;46(2):173–8.

17. Takeshita S, Asano H, Hata T, et al. Comparison of frequency of radial artery occlusion after 4Fr versus 6Fr transradial coronary intervention (from the Novel Angioplasty USIng Coronary Accessor Trial). Am J Cardiol 2014;113(12):1986–9.

18. Dahm JB, Vogelgesang D, Hummel A, et al. A randomized trial of 5 vs. 6 French transradial percutaneous coronary interventions. Catheter Cardiovasc Interv 2002;57(2):172–6.

19. Pancholy S, Coppola J, Patel T, et al. Prevention of radial artery occlusion-patent hemostasis evaluation trial (PROPHET study): a randomized comparison of traditional versus patency documented hemostasis after transradial catheterization. Catheter Cardiovasc Interv 2008;72(3):335–40.

20. Barbeau GR. Evaluation of the ulnopalmar arterial arches with pulse oximetry and plethysmography: comparison with the Allen's test in 1010 patients. Am Heart J 2004;147(3):489–93.

21. Pancholy SB, Patel TM. Effect of duration of hemostatic compression on radial artery occlusion after transradial access. Catheter Cardiovasc Interv 2012;79(1):78–81.

22. Spaulding C, Lefèvre T, Funck F, et al. Left radial approach for coronary angiography: results of a prospective study. Cathet Cardiovasc Diagn 1996; 39(4):365–70.

23. Bertrand OF, Rao SV, Pancholy S, et al. Transradial approach for coronary angiography and interventions: results of the first international transradial practice survey. JACC Cardiovasc Interv 2010; 3(10):1022–31.

24. Pancholy SB. Comparison of the effect of intra-arterial versus intravenous heparin on radial artery occlusion after transradial catheterization. Am J Cardiol 2009;104(8):1083–5.

25. Plante S, Cantor WJ, Goldman L, et al. Comparison of bivalirudin versus heparin on radial artery occlusion after transradial catheterization. Catheter Cardiovasc Interv 2010;76(5):654–8.

26. Feray H, Izgi C, Cetiner D, et al. Effectiveness of enoxaparin for prevention of radial artery occlusion after transradial cardiac catheterization. J Thromb Thrombolysis 2010;29(3):322–5.

27. Pancholy SB, Ahmed I, Bertrand OF, et al. Frequency of radial artery occlusion after transradial access in patients receiving warfarin therapy and undergoing coronary angiography. Am J Cardiol 2014;113(2):211–4.

28. Bernat I, Bertrand OF, Rokyta R, et al. Efficacy and safety of transient ulnar artery compression to recanalize acute radial artery occlusion after transradial catheterization. Am J Cardiol 2011;107(11): 1698–701.

29. Rhyne D, Mann T. Hand ischemia resulting from a transradial intervention: successful management with radial artery angioplasty. Catheter Cardiovasc Interv 2010;76(3):383–6.

30. Ruzsa Z, Pinter L, Kolvenbach R. Anterograde recanalisation of the radial artery followed by transradial angioplasty. Cardiovasc Revasc Med 2010; 11(4):266.e1–4.

31. Babunashvili A, Dundua D. Recanalization and reuse of early occluded radial artery within 6 days after previous transradial diagnostic procedure. Catheter Cardiovasc Interv 2011;77(4):530–6.

32. He GW, Yang CQ. Characteristics of adrenoceptors in the human radial artery: clinical implications. J Thorac Cardiovasc Surg 1998;115(5):1136–41.

33. Jia DA, Zhou YJ, Shi DM, et al. Incidence and predictors of radial artery spasm during transradial coronary angiography and intervention. Chin Med J (Engl) 2010;123(7):843–7.

34. Ruiz-Salmeron RJ, Mora R, Vélez-Gimón M, et al. Radial artery spasm in transradial cardiac catheterization. Assessment of factors related to its occurrence, and of its consequences during follow-up. Rev Esp Cardiol (Engl Ed) 2005;58(5): 504–11.

35. Kiemeneij F, Vajifdar BU, Eccleshall SC, et al. Evaluation of a spasmolytic cocktail to prevent radial artery spasm during coronary procedures. Catheter Cardiovasc Interv 2003;58(3):281–4.

36. Varenne O, Jégou A, Cohen R, et al. Prevention of arterial spasm during percutaneous coronary interventions through radial artery: the SPASM study. Catheter Cardiovasc Interv 2006;68(2):231–5.

37. Rosencher J, Chaïb A, Barbou F, et al. How to limit radial artery spasm during percutaneous coronary interventions: the spasmolytic agents to avoid spasm during transradial percutaneous coronary interventions (SPASM3) study. Catheter Cardiovasc Interv 2013;84:766–71.

38. Rathore S, Stables RH, Pauriah M, et al. Impact of length and hydrophilic coating of the introducer sheath on radial artery spasm during transradial coronary intervention: a randomized study. JACC Cardiovasc Interv 2010;3(5):475–83.

39. Pancholy SB, Karuparthi PR, Gulati R. A novel non-pharmacologic technique to remove entrapped radial sheath. Catheter Cardiovasc Interv 2014;85: E35–8.

40. Pullakhandam NS, Yang ZJ, Thomas S, et al. Unusual complication of transradial catheterization. Anesth Analg 2006;103(3):794–5.

41. Dieter RS, Akef A, Wolff M. Eversion endarterectomy complicating radial artery access for left heart catheterization. Catheter Cardiovasc Interv 2003; 58(4):478–80.

42. Bertrand OF, Larose E, Rodés-Cabau J, et al. Incidence, predictors, and clinical impact of bleeding after transradial coronary stenting and maximal antiplatelet therapy. Am Heart J 2009;157(1): 164–9.

43. Tizon-Marcos H, Barbeau GR. Incidence of compartment syndrome of the arm in a large series of transradial approach for coronary procedures. J Interv Cardiol 2008;21(5):380–4.

44. Tizon-Marcos H, Bertrand OF, Rodés-Cabau J, et al. Impact of female gender and transradial coronary stenting with maximal antiplatelet therapy on bleeding and ischemic outcomes. Am Heart J 2009; 157(4):740–5.

45. Friedrich JB, Shin AY. Management of forearm compartment syndrome. Hand Clin 2007;23(2): 245–54, vii.

46. Bertrand OF. Acute forearm muscle swelling post transradial catheterization and compartment syndrome: prevention is better than treatment! Catheter Cardiovasc Interv 2010;75(3):366–8.

47. Calvino-Santos RA, Vázquez-Rodríguez JM, Salgado-Fernández J, et al. Management of iatrogenic radial artery perforation. Catheter Cardiovasc Interv 2004;61(1):74–8.

48. Sanmartin M, Cuevas D, Goicolea J, et al. Vascular complications associated with radial artery access for cardiac catheterization. Rev Esp Cardiol (Engl Ed) 2004;57(6):581–4.

49. Yokoyama N, Takeshita S, Ochiai M, et al. Anatomic variations of the radial artery in patients undergoing transradial coronary intervention. Catheter Cardiovasc Interv 2000;49(4):357–62.

50. Gunasekaran S, Cherukupalli R. Radial artery perforation and its management during PCI. J Invasive Cardiol 2009;21(2):E24–6.

51. Rigatelli G, Dell'Avvocata F, Ronco F, et al. Successful coronary angioplasty via the radial approach after sealing a radial perforation. JACC Cardiovasc Interv 2009;2(11):1158–9.

52. Narayan RL, Vaishnava P, Kim M. Radial artery perforation during transradial catheterization managed with a coronary polytetrafluoroethylene-covered stent graft. J Invasive Cardiol 2012;24(4): 185–7.

53. Collins N, Wainstein R, Ward M, et al. Pseudoaneurysm after transradial cardiac catheterization: case series and review of the literature. Catheter Cardiovasc Interv 2012;80(2):283–7.

54. Herold J, Brucks S, Boenigk H, et al. Ultrasound guided thrombin injection of pseudoaneurysm of the radial artery after percutaneous coronary intervention. Vasa 2011;40(1):78–81.

55. Liou M, Tung F, Kanei Y, et al. Treatment of radial artery pseudoaneurysm using a novel compression device. J Invasive Cardiol 2010;22(6):293–5.

56. Spence MS, Byrne J, Haegeli L, et al. Rare access site complications following transradial coronary intervention. Can J Cardiol 2009;25(6):e206.

57. Kwac MS, Yoon SJ, Oh SJ, et al. A rare case of radial arteriovenous fistula after coronary angiography. Korean Circ J 2010;40(12):677–9.

58. Pulikal GA, Cox ID, Talwar S. Images in cardiovascular medicine. Radial arteriovenous fistula after cardiac catheterization. Circulation 2005;111(6):e99.

59. Dehghani P, Culig J, Patel D, et al. Arteriovenous fistula as a complication of transradial coronary angiography: a case report. J Med Case Rep 2013;7:21.

60. Papadimos TJ, Hofmann JP. Radial artery thrombosis, palmar arch systolic blood velocities, and

chronic regional pain syndrome 1 following transradial cardiac catheterization. Catheter Cardiovasc Interv 2002;57(4):537–40.

61. Sasano N, Tsuda T, Sasano H, et al. A case of complex regional pain syndrome type II after transradial coronary intervention. J Anesth 2004;18(4):310–2.

62. Cho EJ, Yang JH, Song YB. Type II complex regional pain syndrome of the hand resulting from repeated arterial punctures during transradial coronary intervention. Catheter Cardiovasc Interv 2013;82(4):E465–8.

63. Subramanian R, White CJ, Sternbergh WC 3rd, et al. Nonhealing wound resulting from a foreign-body reaction to a radial arterial sheath. Catheter Cardiovasc Interv 2003;59(2):205–6.

64. Kozak M, Adams DR, Ioffreda MD, et al. Sterile inflammation associated with transradial catheterization and hydrophilic sheaths. Catheter Cardiovasc Interv 2003;59(2):207–13.

65. Zellner C, Ports TA, Yeghiazarians Y, et al. Sterile radial artery granuloma after transradial cardiac catheterization. Cardiovasc Revasc Med 2011; 12(3):187–9.

66. Patel T, Shah S, Pancholy S. A simple approach for the reduction of knotted coronary catheter in the radial artery during the transradial approach. J Invasive Cardiol 2011;23(5):E126–7.

67. Kim JY, Moon KW, Yoo KD. Entrapment of a kinked catheter in the radial artery during transradial coronary angiography. J Invasive Cardiol 2012;24(1):E3–4.

The Transradial Learning Curve and Volume-Outcome Relationship

Ian C. Gilchrist, MD, FSCAI

KEYWORDS

• Cardiac catheterization • Learning curve • Percutaneous coronary intervention

---

KEY POINTS

- Learning curves involving medical procedures are confounded by many known and other poorly recognized factors.
- Despite the limitation in the medical science of learning curves, recent data suggest a learning curve of 30 to 50 cases for transradial interventional procedures.
- Although learning can be measured based on x-ray exposure or contrast use, the metrics of improved patient safety from access site complications or preservation of procedural success seem to have no learning curve.
- Benefits from conversion to transradial from transfemoral catheterization seem to start immediately in the learning process and exist despite differences in volume.

INTRODUCTION

Adoption of transradial technology in the United States during cardiac catheterization has trailed that of many other countries around the world. One of the explanations offered for this lagging transition in the United States has concerned the concept of learning curves and inadequate procedural volume in the United States. In this article these issues are discussed and the present understanding of the evidence explored.

BACKGROUND

Learning curves in health care typically follow a power curve relationship although a wide variety of other relationships are potentially observable.[1] The power curve typically measures an outcome on the y-axis as cumulative experience is documented along the x-axis, as shown in Fig. 1. The learning curve can be used to quantitate the number of procedures needed to start to attain proficiency by statistically defining the point or region of the curve where incremental benefit starts to diminish with each additional

procedure or experience. Although this point should not be considered the true point of mastery, it does seem to indicate an initial level of proficiency in the learning cycle.

DESCRIPTORS OF LEARNING CURVES

The use of the adjective steep, as in steep learning curves, can indicate either a portion of the learning experience in which incremental advancement is large per unit of experience, or may also refer to a learning experience that is long to attain the required proficiency. Therefore, the use of the term steep, or its contrary descriptors, can be confusing and at times inappropriate unless the procedure or outcome is being compared with a known learning curve. A curve is only steep or long when it is comparable with another curve measuring a similar activity.

LEARNING CURVES IN MEDICAL FIELD

The learning curve is conceptually simple and self-evident as an extension of the classic proverb: practice makes perfect. It is the application

---

The author has nothing to disclose.
Division of Cardiology, Heart and Vascular Institute, Pennsylvania State University College of Medicine, 500 University Drive, Hershey, PA 17033, USA
E-mail address: icg1@psu.edu

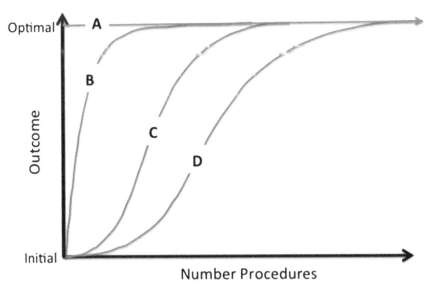

Fig. 1. Typical learning curves plotting increasing number of procedures against outcome. Curve A represents no effective learning curve with advantages of a new procedure instantly available on the switch to new procedure. This curve might be representative of the reduction in access site complication seen immediately on starting radial procedures. Curve B shows a quicker or shorter learning experience versus curve C. Curve D represents a longer learning experience versus curve B, and curve C and represents a steeper or harder learning curve.

of this concept in the medical field and use in the individual physician that presents a variety of issues.

- Medical procedures and treatments are done in an environment with confounders distinctly different from what might be easily controlled on an industrial factory floor.
- Each procedure is performed on different patients with individual characteristics affecting outcome, and different operators with varying background experience and individual learning personalities.
- Each institution where these procedures are performed differs by institutional provisions and variations in support staff capabilities.

CONFOUNDING FACTORS
Variability in Operators
In transradial procedures, the mix of variables to adjust can be daunting. For example, the following considerations are related to operator or physician learners:

- Transradial techniques are new procedures being adopted by operators whose background experience may vary from those fresh from fellowship training to others who have been in practice for multiple decades.

- In measuring outcomes, there is often difficulty in retrospectively defining why the operator chose the patient to undergo the selected procedure verses another approach.
- Operator confidence is difficult to ascertain.

Operator Confidence
An early positive experience on low-risk patients with a new technique could skew the curve if later exuberance causes the operator to take on higher risk patients before the skill set has matured. An example of this phenomenon can be seen in Fig. 2 from the arterial closure litera-ture in which later patients subjected to the pro-cedure were at higher risk for adverse outcome. The net success therefore decreased, at least transiently, while further experience was ac-quired.[2] The reverse is also possible: a lack of confidence despite a reasonable outcome can delay rapid adaption of new skills. Operators starting a new procedure in a nonsupportive environment might experience a delayed learning curve. Some of the delay in transradial adaption in the United States may be considered an example of this phenomenon.

Different Modes of Learning Same New Information
The medical learning environment is difficult to understand and model for understanding.

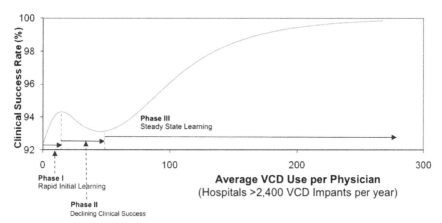

Fig. 2. Triphasic learning curve seen with vascular closure device (VCD). Triphasic learning curves in the largest hospital quartile with annual institutional volume of more than 2400 VCD implants per year. Phase I represents the initial early learning curve. Phase II represents declining success most likely caused by more challenging patients before physician skills are commensurate with the challenge. Phase III represents a later steady state learning curve that continues until the process levels off beyond 200 implants per year. (*From* Resnic FS, Wang TY, Arora N, et al. Quantifying the learning curve in the use of a novel vascular closure device: an analysis of the NCDR (National Cardiovascular Data Registry) CathPCI registry. JACC Cardiovasc Interv 2012;5(1):87; with permission.)

Learning may occur with operators working with a mentor or coach, through applying information learned at a didactic weekend course, or by attempting to self-expand skills based on prior experience and independent education. Not only may the form or conduit of learning be diverse among physicians, there are also personality differences between physicians that may allow some to be more facile at conceptualizing and grasping new procedures.

Early Adopters Versus Followers
Transradial technology was a novel approach when introduced into the femoral-dominated cardiovascular community. Adoption of new technology follows a predictable course that was first noted during the introduction of modern farming practices in the 1950s[3] and popularized in the modern press especially in the spread of high-tech innovations. Innovators and early adopters have distinctly different personality types and characteristics from later adopters. Evaluating learning curves therefore also needs to take into consideration where on the technology adoption cycle the learners are. Because transradial adoption in the United States has only recently become widespread,[4] much of the older US literature reflects activities related to innovators and early adopters rather than the experience of most operators.

Patient and Institutional Variables
Learner variants and confounders are just a few of the issues that are difficult to account for and measure.

- Each patients is unique and outcomes are not perfectly predictable.
- Hospitals have institutional personalities that are variable, ranging from small community facilities to massive academic centers with deeply embedded cultures of learning and investigation.
- Support staffs at different institutions are variable both in skill sets and enthusiasm for changing to or learning new procedures.

Because transradial techniques represent not just a shift in technique but also an opportunity to affect a whole spectrum of health care processes, the acceptance or resistance to adoption by support staff can facilitate or retard the learning process. All of these factors may be difficult to prospectively capture or quantitate, but they are just a few example of possible confounders to understanding the learning curve of radial procedures.

OUTCOME MEASURES: WHAT ARE CLINICIANS LEARNING?

Challenges exist in transradial catheterization to define an outcome suitable for generating a learning curve.

- The outcome has to be common enough to be measurable over a period of dynamic change.
- The outcome has to have some relevance or value as a surrogate for the performance of the procedure.

- Hard end points of death or myocardial infarction are rare in cardiac catheterization and, at least at the individual level, unlikely to resolve the question of proficiency.

Problems with Surrogate Outcomes of Proficiency
Length of procedure
Surrogates such as procedure length, contrast use, or x-ray exposure are easy to measure, but the simplicity raises questions of relevance or adequacy of the measure. For instance, the length of a procedure may be one measure of outcome, but the length of hospitalization (or door-to-door time) may reflect the system's learning curve as a new technology causes adjustment in hospital protocols and care processes. Which results should be considered most relevant if the procedure is slightly longer but the patient is discharged much earlier with a new procedure on the learning curve?

Radiation exposure
Learning curves measuring patient x-ray exposure may follow a different curve than that of operator x-ray exposure and raise an issue of which is more relevant.

- Is it acceptable for a patient to receive more radiation in exchange for a decreased rate of complications?
- How much extra radiation is acceptable for the operator in order to reduce the patient's risk of an adverse outcome?

Some transradial studies may have experienced this issue of relevance, especially when intraoperator variability is much greater than measured differences between techniques.[5,6] More recent studies have suggested little difference in radiation exposure between femoral and radial procedures as long as experience and protection are controlled.[7,8] X-ray exposure is confounded by the problem of poor understanding of x-ray hazards by some physicians and institutional staff resulting in a measure that has diminished relevance to those operators.

Changing best-practice benchmarks
The transradial experience and reporting of learning curves need to be considered critically in the context of the confounded environment on which these studies were based.

- Best practices for transradial procedures continue to evolve.
- Advances in technology, such as the introduction of hydrophilic sheaths and

better catheters, result in a soft basis to define optimal outcome because the frames of reference keep changing.

Outcomes related to radial artery occlusion represent a relevant example. As the understanding of anticoagulation, patent hemostasis, and ability to use small devices grows, the outcome of arterial occlusion changes. Likewise the method and timing used to assess this outcome markedly changes the result.

LEARNING CURVE INVESTIGATIONS
Overview
There has been a variety of studies[9-17] examining the issue of the transradial learning curve from the mid-1990s to 2014. All but the latest, by Hess and colleagues[16] and Gutierrez and colleagues,[17] are:

- Single-center experiences, and limited to some extent by the statistical hazards of low numbers.
- In general lacking clarity from the viewpoint of operator experience and institutional experience.
- Using surrogates such as fluoroscopy times, procedural time in the cardiac catheterization laboratory, or contrast use to measure extent of learning.

Despite these shortcomings, the overall results are consistent, especially considering the diverse nature of institutions reporting from worldwide geographic locations, and the technologic changes in the last 20 years. Using simple measurements of outcome, the number of procedures to become proficient is in the range of 25 to 80 cases. More recent studies favor shorter learning curves, which likely reflects both better technology for transradial access and improved learning resources, including didactic courses and local experience with mentorship.

United States–Based Learning Curves from Registry Data
The recent publication by Hess and colleagues[16] uses data from the CathPCI Registry, which collects data from more than 1400 US hospitals and provides the first broad-based contemporary assessment of the learning curve for transradial percutaneous coronary intervention (PCI) in the United States. They focused their analysis on new radial operators, which was defined for analysis as any registered operators who recorded their first transradial procedure 6 months or greater after their first transfemoral procedure starting on July 1, 2009. Primary

outcomes included median fluoroscopy time, median contrast volume, and procedure success. Secondary end points included in-hospital mortality, vascular complications, access site bleeding, access site hematoma, and any bleeding event. Outcomes were then examined by grouping the operators into 1 of 4 volume strata (1–10 procedures, 11–50 procedures, 51–100 procedures, and 101–200 procedures).

Across the 4 volume strata, there was no significant difference in procedural success.

- Median fluoroscopy time shortened incrementally across each level of case volume with the higher volume operators associated with the lowest times.
- Contrast usage decreased significantly with experience, although most of this decrease was seen within the first 2 groups (1–10 and 11–50 procedures).
- Beginning operators as defined in the study gained their experience without loss of procedure success.
- Vascular complications, access site bleeding, or hematoma was low across all groups.
- Stable success rate remained after adjustment for patient and procedural characteristics, suggesting that as the operators gained experience they maintained their success despite potentially attempting more complex procedures.

Because the net procedural outcome and safety were undifferentiated across the operator volumes, the relationships between procedural volume and the primary outcomes of fluoroscopy time and contrast usage were used to define the learning curve. These knot points or inflection points in the power curves suggested that, for the measures used, between 30 and 50 cases were required to overcome the learning curve.

United States–Based Learning Curves from Veterans Administration Data

An analysis from the US Veterans Administration health system was done by Gutierrez and colleagues,[17] using a group of 24,142 patients undergoing PCI between 2007 and 2010. In the 3 subgroups of institutional volume (≥1 radial PCI, ≥50 radial PCIs, or <50 radial PCIs):

- There was no difference in overall procedural success, transfusion, or mortality.
- In a comparison dichotomizing the institutions at the 50-radial-PCI cut point,

there was an association with a decreased risk of transfusion at the higher volume centers but no difference in risk of mortality.

RELATIONSHIP OF VOLUME AND OUTCOMES

United States General Catheterization Procedure Volume-Outcome Relationship

The analyses of Hess and colleagues[16] and Gutierrez and colleagues[17] show no association between operator radial volume and mortality. The association between PCI volume and mortality has been reported in the past. A contemporary review of the individual and institutional mortality outcome and PCI volume has recently been published using data from 2005 to 2009 in the National Inpatient Sample database of the Healthcare Cost and Utilization Project using a sample of 457,498 procedures.[18] Although this study did not break down outcomes by access site, it is reasonable to assume that, because less than 5% of the procedures recorded in the CathPCI registry over this period were transradial, the results represent a primarily transfemoral outcome. Although it was hoped that procedural improvements might have attenuated or eliminated the earlier reported volume-outcome relationships, this analysis suggests otherwise, because the probability of mortality and periprocedural complications minimized at an annual PCI volume of 300. The question of what role the transradial approach plays in this relationship in the United States has not been addressed in a large enough sample to provide a definitive answer.

International Radial/Femoral Access Procedure Volume-Outcome Relationship

Outside the United States, a volume-outcome relationship has been seen and measured specifically around the issue of transradial and femoral catheterization. The RIVAL (A Trial of Transradial Versus Trans-femoral Percutaneous Coronary Intervention [PCI] Access Site Approach in Patients With Unstable Angina or Myocardial Infarction Managed With an Invasive Strategy) study was a large (N = 7021) randomized trial of transradial or transfemoral catheterization or PCI in patients with acute coronary syndromes. Although the overall study showed no significant difference between a transfemoral or radial approach, a significant interaction between procedural volume and access site was noted.[19]

- In the subgroup with ST segment elevation myocardial infarction (STEMI), transradial catheterization was associated with improved outcome compared with transfemoral catheterization, including lower mortality.

- No association was seen between low-volume, medium-volume, and high-volume operators and their outcomes between transradial or femoral catheterization.
- Multivariable modeling showed an independent association between institutional radial volume and outcome with the sites with higher radial volumes having the better outcomes. This institutional volume effect was not seen in the femoral group.
- There was no association of PCI complications by volume, although there remained a persistent reduction in access site and bleeding complications in the transradial rather than femoral access groups.

This study of Jolly and colleagues[19] suggests that, in a high-volume environment such as is found in the sites used for the RIVAL trial, improvements in outcome continue to accrue as the experience of the operator and institution increase. However, in the United States, most operators would have been classified as low volume because most US operators perform fewer than or equal to 70 radial-PCI/y (median $\leq$60 radial-PCI/operator/y).[20] Without a major disruption of the present US health care system, the institutional volume and individual experience seen elsewhere will not be obtained in the United States.

TRAINING AND INTERACTIONS IN OUTCOME IN THE UNITED STATES

Given the low individual PCI annual volume in the United States, it might be concerning that transition to the transradial approach might be hazardous, with operators never fully surmounting the learning curve. Several investigations have suggested otherwise. These studies involve both the safety of introducing transradial training into US fellowships and the safety of transition to transradial approaches during procedures by experienced practitioners.

Transradial Cardiac Catheterization Training Requirements

The best-practice statement published by the Society for Cardiovascular Angiography and Intervention noted that there are no prescribed approaches to fellowship training for transradial catheterization, but suggested that both transradial and femoral catheterization be introduced in parallel under most circumstances in which appropriate instruction is available.[21] The Accreditation Council for Graduate Medical Education[22] and American College of Cardiology Core Cardiology Training Symposium[23] guidelines both point to the need for knowledge of transradial catheterization in addition to transfemoral techniques, although the execution of these guidelines is left vague. Part of this vagueness on how to meet this training requirement may have stemmed from the lack of general training available across the United States in fellowship programs when these training guidelines were constructed.

OUTCOMES AND INSTITUTIONAL TRANSITION TO TRANSRADIAL CATHETERIZATION

Transitioning in Academic Training Centers

Leonardi and colleagues[24] in 2012 published their experience at a university training program as transradial catheterization was introduced into the program for both attendings and fellows. During a 2-year transition (2008–2010) outcomes were analyzed for procedural success and complications. The results supported a conclusion that transradial programs are likely to improve PCI safety.

- There were no differences in procedural success across the period, although the transradial procedures were noted to require slightly more fluoroscopy time.
- Procedural times and contrast volumes were similar between the radial and femoral procedures.
- As the transition to transradial approach proceeded, the safety outcome of bleeding and vascular complications decreased from 2.0% to 0.7% ($P = .05$) during the 2 year period.

A similar experience was published by Balwanz and colleagues[25] from the University of California as they transitioned from femoral to radial approaches in their fellowship program.

- There was an increase in procedural factors, such as fluoroscopy or procedure duration times, between the radial and femoral angiographic procedures, although this difference did not extend to interventional procedures.
- There was a trend toward less contrast volume in both the transradial and femoral patients in the last half of the transition.
- Procedural success was high in both groups, whereas the transition to the transradial approach reduced the rate of vascular complications.

The investigators hypothesized that the persistence of long fluoroscopy and procedural times for diagnostic cases might represent a longer learning curve for new operators, but, nevertheless, the results were dominated by the increased safety of fewer vascular complications seen throughout the transition.

Fellowship training may offer some advantages to learning the transradial approach, assuming appropriate supervision is available. Most recent medical residency graduates are likely to be more comfortable with establishing radial arterial access than femoral access given the required proficiency with arterial lines for invasive blood pressure monitoring. In addition, they have not been exposed to transfemoral catheterization and therefore both approaches are learned from a common baseline of knowledge without prior practice bias.

Transitioning Previously Femoral-Trained Cardiologists to the Radial Approach

Although fellows-in-training have a blank slate of experience on which to train, seasoned cardiologists may face other challenges based on past practice experiences and willingness to change what they perceive to be an otherwise routine practice strategy. Can those who are already in practice be trained, or is it necessary to wait for time to replace legacy operators with freshly trained graduates? Several studies have provided at least some insight into this question.

Barbash and colleagues,[26] from a well-known cardiovascular center in the United States, published their experience in converting from femoral to transradial practice, which was similar to that reported from fellowship programs

- They experienced an initial increase in fluoroscopy times, although contrast use was less in the transradial group.
- Overall procedural success and long-term outcomes remained the same during the transition.
- The investigators thought that the transition from femoral to radial access occurred with no material learning curve.

A similar study of the effects of transition from femoral to radial approaches was published from a New Zealand hospital where, over a 1-year period, 8 operators performed cardiac catheterization on 1004 patients with or without PCI.[27]

- Procedural success was similar between those initial patients undergoing transfemoral procedures and the later patients undergoing transradial procedures.
- Vascular access site complications decreased from 4.8% in the femoral group to 0.25% in the radial group (P<.0001).

This observation that safety, as manifested by a reduction in vascular access site complications, occurs regardless of the learning curve measure is a recurrent observation in the literature and is a benefit seen essentially from the first radial experience.

SUMMARY/DISCUSSION

Learning curves are pervasive in the modern world. Their usefulness and relevance depend on the measures used and an understanding of the background confounders. The practice of medicine is more complicated than the industrial plants where these concepts first arose and appropriate interpretation requires an understanding of the limitations of the literature.

Transradial catheterization represents a new approach in cardiology that alters the status quo and requires further training for practicing cardiologists to adapt. As this techniques spreads from early adopters and innovators to the general cardiology community, a need to understand the learning curve for this procedural approach exists for professional competency and ensuring patient safety.

Despite the limitations that exist in most of the published experiences that have attempted to resolve the question of the learning curve, there is an overall consistent result over their experiences suggesting a manageable learning curve of fewer than 100 cases. The most recent analysis suggests an experience of 30 to 50 cases on average represents the learning curve based on the metrics of contrast use and fluoroscopy time.

Although the relationship between PCI volumes exists and evidence in patients with STEMI can show improved outcomes in transradial patients done at the highest-volume institutions, there seem to be no safety concerns about transition from femoral to radial approaches. Reduction in the risk of access site complications and bleeding occur from the first transradial patient and transition can occur without measurable difference in procedural outcome and clinical success. These factors are most relevant to transitioning cardiologists and the patients who are subjected to these procedures as their doctors retool for the future.

REFERENCES

1. Ramsay CR, Wallace SA, Garthwaite PH, et al. Assessing the learning curve effect in health technologies. Lessons from the nonclinical literature. Int J Technol Assess Health Care 2002;18(1):1–10.

2. Resnic FS, Wang TY, Arora N, et al. Quantifying the learning curve in the use of a novel vascular closure device: an analysis of the NCDR (National Cardiovascular Data Registry) CathPCI registry. JACC Cardiovasc Interv 2012;5(1):82–9.

3. Subcommittee for the study of Diffusion in Farm Practices. How farm people accept new ideas. North Central Regional Extension Publication No. 1. Special Report No. 15. Ames (IA): Agricultural Extension Service; 1955.

4. Feldman DN, Swaminathan RV, Kaltenbach LA, et al. Adoption of radial access and comparison of outcomes to femoral access in percutaneous coronary intervention: an updated report from the NCDR (2007-2012). Circulation 2013;127:2295–306.

5. Mercuri M, Mehta S, Xie C, et al. Radial artery access as a predictor of increased radiation exposure during a diagnostic cardiac catheterization procedure. JACC Cardiovasc Interv 2011;4(3):347–52.

6. Shah B, Bangalore S, Feit F, et al. Radiation exposure during coronary angiography via transradial or transfemoral approaches when performed by experienced operators. Am Heart J 2013;165(3):286–92.

7. Rigattieri S, Sciahbasi A, Drefahl S, et al. Transradial access and radiation exposure in diagnostic and interventional coronary procedures. J Invasive Cardiol 2014;26(9):469–74.

8. Lo TS, Ratib K, Chong AY, et al. Impact of access site selection and operator expertise on radiation exposure; a controlled prospective study. Am Heart J 2012;164(4):455–61.

9. Goldberg SL, Renslo R, Sinow R, et al. Learning curve in the use of the radial artery as vascular access in the performance of percutaneous transluminal coronary angioplasty. Cathet Cardiovasc Diagn 1998;44(2):147–52.

10. Spaulding C, Lefèvre T, Funck F, et al. Left radial approach for coronary angiography: results of a prospective study. Cathet Cardiovasc Diagn 1996;39(4):365–70.

11. Ball WT, Sharieff W, Jolly SS, et al. Characterization of operator learning curve for transradial coronary interventions. Circ Cardiovasc Interv 2011;4(4):336–41.

12. Looi JL, Cave A, El-Jack S. Learning curve in transradial coronary angiography. Am J Cardiol 2011;108(8):1092–5.

13. Carrillo X, Mauri J, Fernandez-Nofrerias E, et al. Safety and efficacy of transradial access in coronary angiography: 8-year experience. J Invasive Cardiol 2012;24(7):346–51.

14. Kasasbeh ES, Parvez B, Huang RL, et al. Learning curve in transradial cardiac catheterization: procedure-related parameters stratified by operators' transradial volume. J Invasive Cardiol 2012; 24(11):599–604.

15. Burzotta F, Trani C, Mazzari MA, et al. Vascular complications and access crossover in 10,676 transradial percutaneous coronary procedures. Am Heart J 2012;163(2):230–8.

16. Hess CN, Peterson ED, Neely ML, et al. The learning curve for transradial percutaneous coronary intervention among operators in the United States: a study from the National Cardiovascular Data Registry. Circulation 2014;129(22): 2277–86.

17. Gutierrez A, Tsai TT, Stanislawski MA, et al. Adoption of transradial percutaneous coronary intervention and outcomes according to center radial volume in the Veterans Affairs Healthcare system: insights from the Veterans Affairs clinical assessment, reporting, and tracking (CART) program. Circ Cardiovasc Interv 2013;6(4):336–46.

18. Badheka AO, Patel NJ, Grover P, et al. Impact of annual operator and institutional volume on percutaneous coronary intervention outcomes: a 5-year United States experience (2005-2009). Circulation 2014;130(6):1392–406.

19. Jolly SS, Cairns J, Yusuf S, et al, RIVAL Investigators. Procedural volume and outcomes with radial or femoral access for coronary angiography and intervention. J Am Coll Cardiol 2014;63(10):954–63.

20. Maroney J, Khan S, Powell W, et al. Current operator volumes of invasive coronary procedures in Medicare patients: implications for future manpower needs in the catheterization laboratory. Catheter Cardiovasc Interv 2013;81(1):34–9.

21. Caputo RP, Tremmel JA, Rao S, et al. Transradial arterial access for coronary and peripheral procedures: executive summary by the Transradial Committee of the SCAI. Catheter Cardiovasc Interv 2011;78(6):823–39.

22. ACGME program requirements for graduate medical education in interventional cardiology (internal medicine), version July 1, 2012. Available at: https://www.acgme.org/acgmeweb/Portals/0/PFAssets/2013-PR-FAQ-PIF/152_interventional_card_int_med_0713 2013_1-YR.pdf. Accessed September 29, 2014.

23. Jacobs AK, Babb JD, Hirshfeld JW Jr, et al. Task force 3: training in diagnostic and interventional cardiac catheterization endorsed by the Society for Cardiovascular Angiography and Interventions. J Am Coll Cardiol 2008;51:355–61.

24. Leonardi RA, Townsend JC, Bonnema DD, et al. Comparison of percutaneous coronary intervention safety before and during the establishment of a transradial program at a teaching hospital. Am J Cardiol 2012;109(8):1154–9.

25. Balwanz CR, Javed U, Singh GD, et al. Transradial and transfemoral coronary angiography and interventions: 1-year outcomes after initiating the transradial approach in a cardiology training program. Am Heart J 2013;165(3):310–6.
26. Barbash IM, Minha S, Gallino R, et al. Operator learning curve for transradial percutaneous coronary interventions: implications for the initiation of a transradial access program in contemporary US practice. Cardiovasc Revasc Med 2014;15(4):195–9.
27. Nadarasa K, Robertson MC, Wong CK, et al. Rapid cycle change to predominantly radial access coronary angiography and percutaneous coronary intervention: effect on vascular access site complications. Catheter Cardiovasc Interv 2012; 79(4):589–94.

The Transradial Approach and Antithrombotic Therapy: Rationale and Outcomes

Alberto Barria Perez, MD, Goran Rimac, MS,
Guillaume Plourde, MS, Yann Poirier, MS,
Olivier Costerousse, PhD, Olivier F. Bertrand, MD, PhD*

KEYWORDS

- Radial artery occlusion • Percutaneous coronary interventions • Antithrombotic therapy
- Transradial approach

KEY POINTS

- Prevention of radial artery occlusion (RAO) should be part of the quality control of any new radial program.
- The incidence of RAO postcatheterization and interventions should probably be initially determined using the gold standard of echo-duplex and later frequently assessed using the less expensive pulse oximetry technique.
- Any evidence of higher risk of RAO should prompt internal analysis and multidisciplinary mechanisms to reduce the risk.
- The most common consequence of chronic RAO is the inability to reuse the radial artery in case of repeat procedure.

INTRODUCTION

The transradial approach for coronary angiography was initially described by Lucien Campeau[1] in 1989. In the early 1990s, the initial impetus for Ferdinand Kiemeneij to perform transradial coronary stent implantation resulted from his despair after the death of a patient following transfemoral coronary stenting and retroperitoneal bleeding (personal communication). Since the early years, the transradial approach has demonstrated clear-cut advantages over the femoral approach in reducing bleeding and access site complications, and consequently improving patient comfort.[2] The radial artery access route has been rapidly adopted by several catheterization laboratory operators, especially in Europe, probably as a result of the lack of a physician's assistant in charge of postprocedural access site management such as practiced in the US health system.[3] Accumulation of a large amount of evidence-based data has provided a new wealth of information and now there is a large increase in radial-based percutaneous coronary interventions (PCIs) in the United States and worldwide. This article reviews the different antithrombotic strategies for PCI according to the access site and the current evidence to limit ischemic complications as well as to prevent radial artery occlusion (RAO).

ANTITHROMBOTIC THERAPY AND PERCUTANEOUS CORONARY INTERVENTION BY TRANSRADIAL APPROACH

Anticoagulants

Heparin

Unfractionated heparin (UFH) was the only anticoagulant available for years before the

The authors have nothing to disclose.
Quebec Heart-Lung Institute, 2725, Chemin Sainte Foy, Quebec City, Quebec G1V 4G5, Canada
* Corresponding author. Interventional Cardiology Laboratories, Quebec Heart-Lung Institute, 2725, Chemin Sainte Foy, Quebec City, Quebec G1V 4G5, Canada.
E-mail address: Olivier.bertrand@crhl.ulaval.ca

Intervent Cardiol Clin 4 (2015) 213–223
http://dx.doi.org/10.1016/j.iccl.2015.01.002
2211-7458/15/$ – see front matter © 2015 Elsevier Inc. All rights reserved.

development of low-molecular-weight heparin (LMWH) and direct thrombin inhibitors. Moreover, UFH is less expensive than every other anticoagulant, if one considers only the drug cost.[4] Currently, UFH remains the default anticoagulant for PCI in most catheterization laboratories.[5] UFH binds to antithrombin and increases the baseline rate of inhibition of clotting factors.[6] Currently, the recommended UFH dose during PCI is a 50 to 70 IU/kg bolus to achieve an activated clotting time (ACT) of 200 to 250 seconds when a glycoprotein IIb-IIIa inhibitor (GPI) is planned. If no GPI is planned, the bolus dose is 70 to 100 IU/kg to achieve a target ACT of 300 to 350 seconds.[7] In a post hoc analysis of the Early Discharge After Transradial Stenting of Coronary Arteries (EASY) trial, after adjustment for baseline and procedural characteristics, a final ACT value greater than 330 seconds was associated with a 47% relative reduction in myocardial infarction (MI) (odds ratio [OR] 0.53, 95% CI 0.29–0.93, P = .024).

In addition, despite that evidence largely comes from femoral approach procedures, heparin has been adopted for transradial approach in a very similar way.[8] A major difference is diagnostic coronary angiography, which can be performed by femoral approach without anticoagulation. In contrast, intravenous (IV) anticoagulation is mandatory with transradial approach, even for diagnostic cases, to reduce the risks of RAO.[5] Although not yet well-defined, it is usually recommended to use a minimum bolus dose of 70 IU/kg UFH or a fixed bolus of 5000 IU. Importantly, the route of administration (intraarterial or IV) does not seem to play a role in the incidence of RAO.[9] It is worth mentioning that an UFH IV bolus is also required in patients who are anticoagulated on warfarin because higher international normalized ratio does not prevent RAO.[10] No data are yet available on patients referred with the so-called new oral anticoagulants.

Low-molecular-weight heparin
LMWH is a heterogeneous mixture of polysaccharides chains with a mean molecular weight of 5000 d. It binds to antithrombin, accelerating its interaction with thrombin and factor Xa. In comparison with heparin, LMWH confers a greater inhibition of the factor Xa and exerts its principle anticoagulation effect at a higher step in the coagulation cascade. Renal excretion plays an important role in LMWH clearance and increased anticoagulant activity is frequently observed in patients with a creatinine clearance less than 30 to 40 mL/min.[11] The Acute STEMI Treated with primary angioplasty and intravenous enoxaparin

Or UFH to Lower ischemic and bleeding events at short- and Long-term follow-up (ATOLL) trial included subjects with ST-elevation myocardial infarction (STEMI) treated by primary PCI. In this trial, 96% of subjects received aspirin and 93% received clopidogrel loading doses. Transradial approach was used in 68% of cases. The trial compared enoxaparin versus UFH and found a significant reduction of secondary endpoint of death, recurrent MI or acute coronary syndrome (ACS), or urgent revascularization (OR 0.68, CI 95% 0.48–0.97, P = .03).[12] In a post hoc analysis of transradial versus femoral-treated subjects, there was no significant difference in the net clinical benefit or ischemic outcomes between transradial subjects with and without GPI, or transradial versus nontransradial patients with GPI. However, there were significantly fewer major bleeding and blood transfusions in transradial subjects with GPI compared with nontransradial subjects with GPI.[13]

Another randomized open-label trial that compared dalteparin with UFH for non-STEMI patients who were treated by PCI predominately by transradial approach (79%) showed no significant differences in terms of death, MI, bleeding, target lesion revascularization, stent thrombosis, or cardiac injury biomarkers elevation.[14] In the Fifth Organization to Assess Strategies in Ischemic Syndromes (OASIS-V) trial, which compared enoxaparin to fondaparinux in 14,159 ACS subjects undergoing angiography (and 7885 undergoing PCI), Hamon and colleagues[15] found that the primary outcome, including death, MI, and refractory ischemia, were similar at 9 days in the transradial and femoral groups (7.1% and 7.7%, respectively). Furthermore, the rates of major bleeding were markedly reduced with fondaparinux compared with enoxaparin for both access sites, from 4.8% to 2.3% (hazard ratio [HR] 0.48, 95% CI 0.37–0.62, P<.0001) for femoral and from 2.4% to 0.9% (HR 0.36, 95% CI 0.11–1.16, P<.08) for transradial.[16]

In light of current evidence, LMWH is at least a noninferior option compared with UFH for PCI by transradial approach. In one mechanistic study, Feray and colleagues[17] reported using a single 60 mg enoxaparin bolus dose through the arterial radial sheath (6Fr) for elective procedures and the investigators reported a 4% RAO at 1 week using Doppler assessment. Thus, RAO incidence with LMWH seems in the same range as values reported with UFH.

Despite the widespread use of UFH for PCI, several limitations should be mentioned. There is an unpredictable anticoagulant response requiring close monitoring. It assembles with antithrombin III to inhibit thrombin and the heparin antithrombin complex cannot inhibit factor Xa, which could promote thrombus growth. Heparin is neutralized by platelet factor IV and von Willebrand multimers, heparin binds to glycoprotein IIb-IIIa receptors, which results in undesirable platelet activation.[4] Finally, heparin use is associated with a risk of heparin-induced thrombocytopenia, which can provoke serious venous and arterial thrombosis.[18,19] These heparin disadvantages have lead to research for alternatives such as bivalirudin, a direct antithrombin agent for preferred use during PCI.

Direct thrombin inhibitors (endovenous)
This class of anticoagulants acts by binding directly within the active site of thrombin, preventing its interaction with substrates that promote coagulation. Bivalirudin is a 20-amino acid peptide that inhibits thrombin by binding to both its active site and anion exosite.[19,20] Another endovenous direct thrombin inhibitor currently in use is argatroban, which has been evaluated mainly in PCI for non-ACS.[21]

Bivalirudin Advantages
The major potential advantage of bivalirudin over UFH seems to be a reduction in peri-PCI bleeding. However, it should be noted, almost all evidence gathered in clinical trials or observational studies with bivalirudin originated from subjects undergoing transfemoral PCI. Furthermore, most studies compared bivalirudin with heparin combined with GPI.

The Acute Catheterization and Urgent Intervention Triage strategy (ACUITY) trial included moderate-risk to high-risk ACS subjects and compared 3 strategies: UFH plus GPI, bivalirudin plus GPI, and bivalirudin alone in subjects who underwent coronary angiography within 72 hours after randomization. There were no relevant differences in composite ischemic endpoints. On the contrary, the investigators evidenced a 50% relative risk reduction for major bleeding in bivalirudin arm versus bivalirudin plus GPI (P = .001) and a 43% relative risk reduction versus heparin plus GPI (P = .001). This difference was due to access site, retroperitoneal, and unknown bleeding.[22] Interestingly, a subanalysis of the ACUITY trial according to transradial versus femoral approach did not suggest significant benefit of bivalirudin in terms of access site bleeding or nonaccess site bleeding in the radial subset.[23] Yet, in both groups, there was almost 45% reduction in the risk of organ bleeding. This observation led to the design and implementation of the ongoing EASY-B2B

trial (NCT01084993). In EASY-B2B, patients at high risk of nonaccess site bleeding are randomized to transradial PCI with UFH monotherapy or bivalirudin. So far, 50% of the intended sample size (n = 2500) has been randomized in Canada and the United States.

The Harmonizing Outcomes With Revascular-iZatiON and Stents in Acute Myocardial Infarction (HORIZONS-AMI) trial evaluated bivalirudin versus UFH plus GPI in STEMI subjects who underwent primary PCI with baseline antiplatelet therapy involving aspirin and clopidogrel. The bivalirudin arm showed 38% relative risk reduction of thrombolysis in myocardial infarction (TIMI) major bleeding (P = .02) and 32% relative risk reduction of cardiac death (P = .045). In addition, the bivalirudin group had lower thrombocytopenia incidence compared with UFH.[24] In a post hoc analysis according to access sites, Généreux and colleagues[25] found that transradial compared with femoral access was associated with significantly lower 30-day rates of a major adverse cardiac event (MACE) (2.0% vs 5.6%, OR 0.35, 95% CI 0.13–0.95, P = .02) and non–coronary artery bypass graft (non-CABG)–related bleeding (3.5% vs 7.6%, OR 0.45, 95% CI 0.21–0.95, P = .03). Regarding non-CABG–related major bleeding, there was a gradual increase from 2.9% in the transradial plus bivalirudin subgroup, to 4.1% in the transradial plus UFH-GPI group, to 5.6% in the femoral plus bivalirudin group, and 9.7% in the femoral plus UFH-GPI subgroup (P<.0001). At 1 year, ischemic and bleeding outcomes were still significantly better with the transradial approach compared with the transfemoral approach.

Due to long-known additional risk of bleeding with GPI, Bertrand and colleagues[26] performed a systematic review and meta-analysis of randomized trials (n = 3) and clinical studies (n = 13) comparing UFH monotherapy with bivalirudin. Overall, they found a substantial 45% relative decrease in major bleeding (OR 0.55, 95% CI 0.43–0.72, P<.0001) with bivalirudin in patients undergoing femoral PCI. Interestingly, a trend toward a possible reduction in early mortality was also observed.

In the recently completed European Ambulance Acute Coronary Syndrome Angiography (EUROMAX) trial, STEMI subjects underwent primary PCI and were randomized to bivalirudin versus UFH. The use of GPI was liberal (11% in the bivalirudin group vs 69% in the heparin group) and 47% of cases were treated by transradial approach. The primary outcome of death or major bleeding occurred in 5.1% of subjects in the bivalirudin group versus 8.5% in the UFH group (P = .001). These benefits were consistent across various subgroups but stemmed from a substantial reduction in major bleeding (2.6% vs 6.0% in the bivalirudin and UFH group, respectively, P = .001).[27] Importantly, the initial message of mortality reduction associated with bivalirudin found in the HORIZON trial was not replicated in this contemporary trial. Again, additional benefit for transradial approach was found in a post hoc subanalysis.[28]

Recently, 3 randomized trials, which compared bivalirudin with UFH monotherapy were presented and highly debated: Novel Approaches in Preventing or Limiting Event III (NAPLES III), How Effective are Antithrombotic Therapies in Primary Percutaneous Coronary Intervention (HEAT-PPCI), and BivaliRudin in Acute MI vs GPI and Heparin Trial (BRIGHT). The latter 2 trials included subjects who underwent PCI, mostly by transradial approach. HEAT-PPCI was a single-center United Kingdom-based randomized trial, which compared bivalirudin versus UFH in STEMI subjects. Eighty percent of primary PCI were done by transradial approach. Surprisingly, at 28-day follow-up, the investigators reported a 52% increase in relative risk for primary outcome of death, new MI, additional revascularization, and cerebrovascular accident (95% CI 1.09–2.13, P = .01) in the bivalirudin arm compared with UFH. This was mainly explained by a higher incidence of definitive stent thrombosis, an ischemic risk already identified in previous trials. Interestingly, no benefit with bivalirudin in terms of rate of major bleeding was found.[29] This trial has generated intense debate because it basically contradicted a decade of positive trials with bivalirudin.[30] It should be noted that in the HEAT-PPCI trial most subjects had an extremely short door-to-balloon time, which precluded any UFH bolus administered in the emergency ward. Radial access was the preferred route, GPI were used only as bailout, and ticagrelor was the default oral antiplatelet agent.

BRIGHT was a randomized multicenter trial performed in 82 hospitals in China. It included subjects with non-STEMI and STEMI who were treated by urgent PCI. Subjects were randomized to 3 strategies: bivalirudin, UFH (100 IU/Kg), or UFH plus GPI (UFH 60 IU/Kg with tirofiban up to 36 hours after PCI). Almost 80% of cases were treated by transradial approach. At 30-day follow-up, bleeding (Bleeding Academic Research Consortium 2–5 definition) was 1.2% in the bivalirudin group versus 3.6% in the UFH group (P = .003) and 5.1% in the UFH plus GPI group (P = .001). There were no significant differences regarding the combined ischemic outcomes: death, MI, ischemia-driven target vessel revascularization, and stroke.[31]

In the NAPLES III trial, presented during the last American College of Cardiology LBCT (Washington, March 29, 2014), subjects at high risk of bleeding according to the Nikolsky score were randomized to bivalirudin or UFH with bailout GPI. All 837 subjects underwent transfemoral PCI. The primary endpoint of in-hospital major bleeding according to Randomized Evaluation in Percutaneous Coronary Intervention Linking Angiomax to Reduced Clinical Events (REPLACE)-2 classification was similar between the bivalirudin arm and the UFH arm (3.3% vs 2.6%, OR 1.28, 95% CI 0.58–2.60, P = .54). Interestingly, there was trend for higher access site bleeding requiring intervention with bivalirudin (1.7% vs 0.5%, P = .1) but clinically overt bleeding with a hemoglobin drop greater than 3 g/dL was lower (0.2% vs 1.4%) with bivalirudin. The use of different bleeding definitions did not alter the results. At 30 days, the rate of MACE was similar in both groups (6.5% vs 4.3%, P = .17) and the rate of stent thrombosis was identical (0.5%) in both groups. Similar outcomes were sustained in both groups up to 1 year after PCI.

Two recent updated meta-analyses comparing bivalirudin to UFH, including the most recent randomized trials (of note, neither BRIGHT nor NAPLES-III have yet been published in peer-review journals), have concluded that no benefit in terms of mortality was associated with bivalirudin, yet a significantly higher risk of stent thrombosis was definitively present. Overall, the benefit for a reduction is greatly reduced when UFH dosing is controlled, GPIs are used only as bail-out therapy, and transradial access is preferred.[31,32] Two large ongoing randomized trials should further shed light on these complex results. The Minimizing Adverse Haemorrhagic Events by TRansradial Access Site and Systemic Implementation of angioX (MATRIX; NCT01433627) trial will be performed in Italy and will include more than 5000 subjects with various randomizations (transradial vs femoral, bivalirudin, UFH with provisional GPI, postprimary PCI infusion of bivalirudin vs none). Results should be available in 2015. In the Safety and Efficacy of Femoral Access vs Radial for Primary Percutaneous Coronary Intervention in ST-Elevation Myocardial Infarction (SAFARI-STEMI; NCT01398254) trial, STEMI patients are randomized to transradial versus femoral approach on a background of bivalirudin.

Antiplatelets

Aspirin

Aspirin remains the mainstay treatment of patients who have been diagnosed with ACS, have faced a major atherothrombotic event, or have moderate-to-high risk for cardiovascular events.[24,33,34] Trials that have explored bivalirudin therapy have always included subjects undergoing aspirin treatment.[35] The latest guidelines recommend an 80 to 160 mg dose.[36] Higher aspirin doses have been reported to increase the bleeding risk without preventing additional cerebrovascular events. Interestingly, in the trial, A Clinical Study Comparing Two Forms of Anti-platelet Therapy After Stent Implantation (GLOBAL-LEADERS, NCT01813435), subjects will be randomized at 1 month after PCI under bivalirudin and with BioMatrix stents (Biosensors, Morges, Switzerland) to ticagrelor monotherapy or standard aspirin plus clopidogrel.

Thienopyridines

The Clopidogrel in Unstable Angina to Prevent Recurrent Events (CURE) trial was done in an ACS setting. It compared clopidogrel versus placebo in addition to aspirin, showing a significant reduction of 20% relative risk for nonfatal MI, stroke, or death for cardiovascular causes.[37] The CURE-PCI substudy, which includes only subjects who underwent PCI, showed a significant benefit in terms of cardiovascular death, MI, or any revascularization (relative risk 0.70, 95% CI 0.50–0.97) in the clopidogrel plus aspirin arm versus aspirin alone.[38] After CURE-PCI, several trials have confirmed the benefit for dual antiplatelet pretreatment before PCI for preventing stent thrombosis.[38,39] It should be noted that subjects waited several days before undergoing PCI, hence a long period was allowed so that a plateau effect of clopidogrel-induced platelet ADP-receptor blockade could be reached. Clinical benefit of clopidogrel pretreatment in reducing the risks of ischemic outcomes was also shown in the Clopidogrel for the Reduction of Events During Observation (CREDO) trial, provided that a 18- to 24-hour time window was reached before PCI.[40] However, since the results of A Comparison of Prasugrel at PCI or Time of Diagnosis of Non–ST-Elevation Myocardial Infarction (ACCOAST) trial were released, the benefit of dual antiplatelet therapy has been largely questioned. In fact, outside patients en route for primary PCI, there is little evidence to suggest that systematic loading with oral antiplatelet agents should be routinely performed.[41]

Currently, efforts have been focused in designing drugs with greater antiplatelet effect than clopidogrel. The TRial to assess Improvement in Therapeutic Outcomes by optimizing platelet inhibitioN with prasugrel—Thrombolysis In Myocardial Infarction 38 (TRITON-TIMI38), a randomized multicenter trial, compared prasugrel with clopidogrel in ACS subjects with TIMI risk score greater than 3 and treated by PCI. The incidence for primary efficacy endpoint at 15 months (death from cardiovascular causes, nonfatal MI, and nonfatal stroke) was 9.9% in the prasugrel arm versus 12.1% in clopidogrel arm (P = .001). This difference was largely related to a significant MI reduction in the prasugrel arm (HR 0.76, 95% CI 0.67–0.85, P<.0001), which accounted for periprocedural and spontaneous MI.[42] A subanalysis from TRITON-TIMI 38 evaluated bleeding outcomes in a subgroup of subjects who underwent PCI by femoral approach versus a radial approach. Incidence of TIMI major and minor bleeding were 1.7% for femoral versus 0.6% for transradial approach (HR 3.09, P = .004). Transfusion was required in 3.6% for femoral versus 1.8% for radial approach subgroup (HR 2.05, P = .002).[43]

The PLATelet inhibition and patient Outcomes (PLATO) trial also included ACS patients with or without ST-segment elevation who were randomly assigned to ticagrelor or clopidogrel in a double-dummy fashion. At 12-months follow-up, an absolute 1.1% decrease in MI in the ticagrelor group (HR 0.84, 95% CI 0.75–0.95, P = .005) was noted, as well as a 1.1% decrease in death from any cause (HR 0.78, 95% CI 0.69–0.89, P<.001) and a 1.1% reduction in stent thrombosis (HR 0.77, 95% CI 0.62–0.95, P = .01).[44] A US and European guidelines committee evaluated this evidence and incorporated both antiplatelet agents as a Class I indication[45] for ACS treatment. Some groups have elected prasugrel or ticagrelor as the default therapy in combination with aspirin.[46]

On behalf of the ACCOAST investigators, Italo Porto recently presented the results according to the access site (LBCT, AIM-RADIAL, Chicago, October 2014). Propensity score analysis was performed because non-STEMI patients in the overall and PCI populations had higher scores using criteria from Can Rapid Risk Stratification of Unstable Angina Patients Suppress Adverse Outcomes with Early Implementation of the ACC/AHA Guidelines (CRUSADE) and Global Registry of Acute Coronary Events (GRACE). Overall, the rate of non-CABG TIMI major and minor bleeding was significantly higher in the overall cohort (HR 3.25, 95% CI 1.80–5.88, P<.001) and in the PCI cohort (HR 3.96, 95% CI 1.93–8.12, P<.001).

Glycoprotein IIb-IIIa receptor inhibitors
Platelet aggregation determined by crosslink of fibrinogen and von Willebrand factor after exposure to IIb-IIIa, is key in thrombus formation. Therefore, strategies inhibiting this final common pathway using a GPI are appealing to minimize the thrombotic risk in patients with ACS.[47] Recent GPI trials have not shown any benefit over dual antiplatelet therapy for PCI in stable coronary disease.[48] Bosch and colleagues[49] recently performed an extensive systematic review and meta-analysis for the Cochrane group and concluded that during PCI (48 trials with 33,513 subjects) GPI reduced all-cause mortality at 30 days (OR 0.79, 95% CI 0.64–0.97) but not at 6 months (OR 0.90, 95% CI 0.77–1.05). However, the combined ischemic endpoint of death-MI was significantly reduced at 30 days (OR 0.66, 95% CI 0.60–0.72) and at 6 months (OR 0.75, 95% CI 0.64–0.86) but at the expense of significantly higher risk of severe bleeding (OR 1.39, 95% CI 1.21–1.61) with an absolute risk increase of 8.0 per 1000 treated subjects.

Taking into consideration this evidence, the latest guidelines recommend GPI for provisional use according to coronary angiography findings for the highest risk ACS patients.[45] Again, most of the evidence supporting GPI use in ACS came from trials that used femoral access as the default approach. Hence, the increased risk of bleeding of GPI paralleled increased awareness of detrimental impact of bleeding on outcomes. Meanwhile, GPI has been evaluated in studies involving transradial approach. A vascular substudy, The comPaRison of Early invasive and conservative treatment in patients with non–ST-elevatiOn Acute Coronary Syndromes (PRES-TO-ACS), compared transradial with femoral approach in high-risk ACS subjects. Use of thienopyridines and GPI was significantly more frequent in the transradial approach cases, yet this group had a 0.7% incidence of in-hospital bleeding versus 2.5% in the femoral group (*P* = .05).[50] A large prospective registry from University Health Network at Toronto evaluated the safety of 10,285 PCI cases by femoral approach versus 3214 cases by transradial approach between 2000 and 2006. GPI was used in 83% of cases. The incidence of access site complications was 2.1% in the femoral versus 0.6% in the transradial group (*P* = .01) and there was 1.4% versus 0.6% bleeding incidence, respectively (*P* = .01).[51] Finally, the ATOLL trial, randomized 910 STEMI subjects to UFH versus LMWH during PCI. The global rate for GPI use was 80%, and 67% of cases

underwent transradial PCI. Major bleeding was 4% in the transradial group versus 9% in the femoral group (*P* = .02). However, there was no significant difference in major bleeding in subjects who were treated or not treated with GPI and were treated by transradial approach.[52] In conclusion, in cases when GPI is considered an option, the transradial approach is particularly appealing because it dramatically reduces the additional bleeding risk of GPI. Despite an overall reduction, GPIs are still commonly used in about 40% of the cases in which STEMI patients undergo primary PCI in the United States and in other countries. In the ST-elevation myocardial infarction treated by RADIAL or femoral approach (STEMI-RADIAL) trial, GPI was used in 45% of subjects in both transradial and femoral groups. Major bleeding and vascular complications were significantly lower in the transradial group compared with the femoral group (1.4% vs 7.2%; *P* = .0001).[53]

OPTIMAL RADIAL HEMOSTASIS AND PREVENTION OF COMPLICATIONS

Obtaining hemostasis after transradial approach coronary angiography or PCI is easier and safer compared with femoral approach.[54] Nevertheless, transradial is not free of complications.[55] Yet, most complications relate to hematoma and very rarely require surgical intervention. A dedicated hematoma scale has been developed for hematoma grading (**Fig. 1**).[56] It might be important to detect and treat aggressively hematoma because compartment syndrome may ensue if forearm hematoma is left untreated for a few hours.[57] It would be highly regrettable that with the rapid growth of transradial approach all over the world, previous experience is neglected and that new reports of compartment syndromes and surgical fasciotomy are published. It can never be repeated enough that this dreadful complication is highly preventable and that radial or ulnar access site management requires a close collaboration between physicians, the catheterization laboratory staff, and the nursing team taking care of the patient on the ward. As discussed above, the incidence of low-grade hematoma is slightly higher when GPI are used but there is no evidence that the incidence of hematoma varies according to other antithrombotic therapies. As a rule, if hematoma or muscle pain and swelling develop during the hemostasis phase, it is recommended to immediately stop GPI infusion and control the level of anticoagulation if heparin or bivalirudin

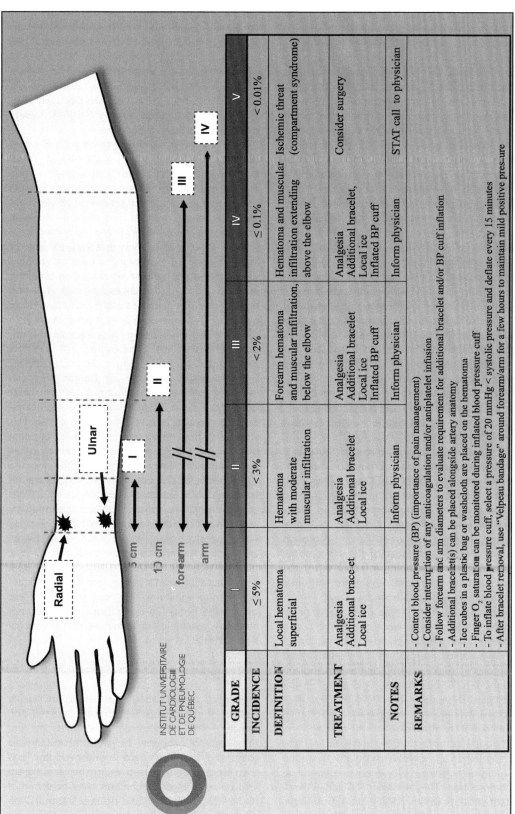

Fig. 1. EASY hematoma classification after transradial/ulnar PCI. (*From* Bertrand OF. Acute forearm muscle swelling post transradial catheterization and compartment syndrome: prevention is better than treatment! Catheter Cardiovasc Interv 2010;75:366–68; with permission.)

drips are used. Currently, there is no evidence to suggest that the incidence of hematoma varies between the use of UFH, LMWH or bivalirudin.

The other most frequent complication is post-procedural RAO. This is often called the Achilles heel of the transradial approach. Since the early days of transradial catheterization, RAO incidence has been reported around 5% when adequate anticoagulation with UFH was provided.[5] However, a review of RAO incidence according to hemostasis techniques and methods of detection suggests that very large variability of RAO exists in everyday practice. In contrast, RAO when no prophylactic anticoagulation was provided has been reported in the 50% to 70% range.[58] Using conventional hemostasis with HemoBand (HemoBand Corp, Portland, OR, USA), no significant difference in RAO between UFH and bivalirudin was found.[59] It should also be noted that spontaneous recanalization might occur over time, hence lessening the rate of RAO. Precise timing is still unknown but it is estimated that 1 to 3 months are necessary before normal radial flow is restored. In an observational study of 563 subjects using 6F introducers and UFH dose between 5000 and 10,000 IU, RAO was 5.3% at discharge from hospital and 2.8% at 1 month as evaluated by echo-duplex.[60]

Apart from anticoagulation, the 2 most important parameters to avoid RAO are (1) the use of smaller catheters,[61] because there is a direct relationship between artery and catheter mismatch and the risk of RAO, and (2) the use of patent hemostasis, which means maintaining radial artery flow during hemostasis. In some studies, subjects pretreated with oral antiplatelet agents had less risk of RAO.[62,63] Although RAO is asymptomatic most of the time, some patients might still complain of arm numbness or local pain, which might require nonsteroidal anti-inflammatory agents for a few days.

The technique for patent hemostasis originated from the seminal work of Cubero[62] and Sanmartin[63] who showed the detrimental impact of crushing and interrupting the radial blood flow on the incidence of RAO. In the randomized Prevention of Radial Artery Occlusion, Patent Hemostasis Evaluation Trial (PROPHET), Pancholy and colleagues[64] compared a traditional 2-hour radial compression to a graded and softer radial compression in which radial flow was maintained as assessed regularly by monitoring digital pulse oximetry during ipsilateral ulnar compression. They obtained 1.8% RAO with a patent strategy versus 7% RAO with traditional hold at 30 days and there was no difference in bleeding. Politi and colleagues[65] attempted to achieve patent hemostasis by applying a nonwoven kaolin-filled pad as an adjunct to manual compression in the puncture site. They compared a short compression (15 minutes) with this pad to a conventional 2-hour compression with a folded sterile gauze, obtaining 0% versus 10% RAO ($P = .05$), respectively, but 20% versus 2% active bleeding ($P<.001$), respectively, after compression.

Patent hemostasis seems the most important technical parameter to avoid acute RAO. Recently, Pancholy and colleagues[66] have demonstrated that IV anticoagulation can be omitted if patent hemostasis can be obtained after radial sheath removal. This could be useful in case the operator would prefer to refrain from providing anticoagulation (trauma patient or active bleeding). However, it must be emphasized that patent hemostasis cannot be obtained in about 25% of the cases because reducing radial pressure immediately induces local bleeding. Implementing patent hemostasis protocol can be challenging because nurses traditionally would not compromise the invisible RAO to oozing or bleeding during hemostasis.

Interestingly, a study by Bernat and colleagues[67] showed that compressing the ulnar artery for 1 hour if RAO is noted could recanalize the radial artery in 71% of the cases. This study was performed with UFH-based anticoagulation and it is not known whether other antithrombotic therapies might influence the success rate of this nonpharmacological way of treating RAO. Some experience using LMWH to treat RAO has been reported, although its real clinical benefit remains unknown because no comparison has been performed between antithrombotic agents to recanalize RAO.[68] It must be emphasized that patients who are anticoagulated on warfarin still require IV anticoagulation to minimize the risks or RAO.[10] No data with so-called new anticoagulants are currently available as a means to prevent or treat RAO.

SUMMARY

Prevention of RAO should be part of the quality control of any new radial program and the incidence of RAO postcatheterization and interventions should probably be determined initially using the gold standard of echo-duplex and then frequently assessed using the less expensive pulse oximetry technique. Any evidence of higher risk of RAO should prompt internal analysis and multidisciplinary mechanisms to be put in place to reduce the risks of RAO. The most common consequence of chronic RAO is the inability to reuse the radial artery in case of repeat procedure.[69]

REFERENCES

1. Campeau L. Percutaneous radial artery approach for coronary angiography. Cathet Cardiovasc Diagn 1989;16:3–7.

2. Kiemeneij F, Laarman GJ, de Melker E. Transradial artery coronary angioplasty. Am Heart J 1995;129(1):1–7.

3. Olivecrona G. Lower mortality with transradial PCI compared to transfemoral PCI in 14,000 patients with acute myocardial infarction: results from SCAAR database. Presented at: EuroPCR. Paris, France, May 20, 2011.

4. Thompson KA, Philip KJ, Schwarz ER. Clinical applications of bivalirudin in the cardiac catheterization laboratory. J Cardiovasc Pharmacol Ther 2011;16(2):140–9.

5. Rao SV, Tremmel JA, Gilchrist IC, et al. Best practices for transradial angiography and intervention: a consensus statement from the society for cardiovascular angiography and intervention's transradial working group. Catheter Cardiovasc Interv 2014;83(2):228–36.

6. Bassand JP. Current antithrombotic agents for acute coronary syndromes: focus on bleeding risk. Int J Cardiol 2013;163(1):5–18.

7. Wright RS, Anderson JL, Adams CD, et al. 2011 ACCF/AHA Focused Update of the Guidelines for the Management of Patients With Unstable Angina/Non-ST-Elevation Myocardial Infarction (Updating the 2007 Guideline): a report of the American College of Cardiology Foundation/American Heart Association Task Force on Practice Guidelines. Circulation 2011;123(18):2022–60.

8. Hamon M, Pristipino C, Di Mario C, et al. Consensus document on the radial approach in percutaneous cardiovascular interventions: position paper by the European Association of Percutaneous Cardiovascular Interventions and Working Groups on Acute Cardiac Care** and Thrombosis of the European Society of Cardiology. EuroIntervention 2013;8(11):1242–51.

9. Pancholy SB. Comparison of the effect of intra-arterial versus intravenous heparin on radial artery occlusion after transradial catheterization. Am J Cardiol 2009;104(8):1083–5.

10. Pancholy SB, Ahmed I, Bertrand OF, et al. Frequency of radial artery occlusion after transradial access in patients receiving warfarin therapy and undergoing coronary angiography. Am J Cardiol 2014;113(2):211–4.

11. Levine GN, Berger PB, Cohen DJ, et al. Newer pharmacotherapy in patients undergoing percutaneous coronary interventions: a guide for pharmacists and other health care professionals. Pharmacotherapy 2006;26(11):1537–56.

12. Montalescot G, Zeymer U, Silvain J, et al. Intravenous enoxaparin or unfractionated heparin in primary percutaneous coronary intervention for ST-elevation myocardial infarction: the international randomised open-label ATOLL trial. Lancet 2011;378(9792):693–703.

13. Iqbal MB, Arujuna A, Ilsley C, et al. Radial versus femoral access is associated with reduced complications and mortality in patients with non-ST-segment-elevation myocardial infarction: an observational cohort study of 10,095 patients. Circ Cardiovasc Interv 2014;7:456–64.

14. Zhang G, Cui W, Li Y, et al. The effect of dalteparin versus unfractionated heparin on the levels of troponin I and creatine kinase isoenzyme MB in elective percutaneous coronary intervention: a multicenter study. Coron Artery Dis 2014;25:510–5.

15. Hamon M, Mehta S, Steg PG, et al. Impact of transradial and transfemoral coronary interventions on bleeding and net adverse clinical events in acute coronary syndromes. EuroIntervention 2011;7(1):91–7.

16. Jolly SS, Faxon D, Fox K, et al. Efficacy and safety of fondaparinux versus enoxaparin in patients with acute coronary syndromes treated with glycoprotein iib/iiia inhibitors or thienopyridines results from the OASIS 5 (Fifth Organization to Assess Strategies in Ischemic Syndromes) trial. J Am Coll Cardiol 2009;54:468–76.

17. Feray H, Izgi C, Cetiner D, et al. Effectiveness of enoxaparin for prevention of radial artery occlusion after transradial cardiac catheterization. J Thromb Thrombolysis 2010;29:322–5.

18. Foo S, Everett B, Yeh R, et al. Prevalence of heparin-induced thrombocytopenia in patients undergoing cardiac catheterization. Am Heart J 2006;1(52):290.e1–7.

19. Crespo E, Oliveira G, Honeycutt E, et al. Evaluation and management of thrombocytopenia and suspected heparin-induced thrombocytopenia in hospitalized patients: the Complications After Thrombocytopenia Caused by Heparin (CATCH) registry. Am Heart J 2009;157:651–7.

20. DeServi S, Mariani G, Mariani M, et al. The bivalirudin paradox: high evidence, low use. J Cardiovasc Med (Hagerstown) 2013;14:334–41.

21. Rössig L, Genth-Zotz S, Rau M, et al. Argatroban for elective percutaneous coronary intervention: the ARG-E04 multi-center study. Int J Cardiol 2011;148:214–9.

22. Stone G, White H, Ohman M, et al. Bivalirudin in patients with acute coronary syndromes undergoing percutaneous coronary intervention: a subgroup analysis from the Acute Catheterization

and Urgent Intervention Triage strategy (ACUITY) trial. Lancet 2007;369(9565):907–19.

23. Hamon M, Rasmussen L, Manoukian S, et al. Choice of arterial access site and outcomes in patients with acute coronary syndromes managed with an early invasive strategy: the ACUITY trial. EuroIntervention 2009;5:115–20.

24. Stone G, Witzenbichler B, Guagliumi G, et al. Bivalirudin during primary PCI in acute myocardial infarction. N Engl J Med 2008;358:2218–30.

25. Généreux P, Mehran R, Palmerini T, et al. Radial access in patients with ST-segment elevation myocardial infarction undergoing primary angioplasty in acute myocardial infarction: the HORIZONS-AMI trial. EuroIntervention 2011;7(8):905–16.

26. Bertrand OF, Belisle P, Joyal D, et al. Comparison of transradial and femoral approaches for percutaneous coronary interventions: a systematic review and hierarchical Bayesian meta-analysis. Am Heart J 2012;163:632–48.

27. Steg G, Van't Hof A, Hamm C, et al. Bivalirudin started during emergency transport for primary PCI. N Engl J Med 2013;369(23):2207–17.

28. Zeymer U, Van't Hof A, Adgey J, et al. Bivalirudin is superior to heparins alone with bailout GP IIb/IIIa inhibitors in patients with ST-segment elevation myocardial infarction transported emergently for primary percutaneous coronary intervention: a pre-specified analysis from the EUROMAX trial. Eur Heart J 2014;21(35):2460–7.

29. Shahzad AK, Kemp I, Mars C, et al. Unfractionated heparin versus bivalirudin in primary percutaneous coronary intervention (HEAT-PPCI): an open-label, single centre, randomised controlled trial. Lancet 2014;384(9957):1849–58.

30. Berger PB, Blankenship JC. Is the heat on HEAT-PPCI appropriate? Lancet 2014;384(9957):1824–6.

31. Cassese S, Byrne RA, Laugwitz KL, et al. Bivalirudin versus heparin in patients treated with percutaneous coronary intervention: a meta-analysis of randomised trials. EuroIntervention 2014. [Epub ahead of print].

32. Cavender M, Sabatine M. Bivalirudin versus heparin in patients planned for percutaneous coronary intervention: a meta-analysis of randomised controlled trials. Lancet 2014;384:599–606.

33. Randomized trial of intravenous streptokinase, oral aspirin, both, or neither among 17,187 cases of suspected acute myocardial infarction: ISIS-2. Lancet 1988;13(2):349–60.

34. Shelton R, Eftychiou C, Somers K, et al. Bivalirudin in patients undergoing primary percutaneous coronary intervention for acute ST-elevation myocardial infarction: outcomes in a large real-world population. EuroIntervention 2013;9(1):118–24.

35. Lincoff AM, Bittl JA, Harrington RA, et al. Bivalirudin and provisional glycoprotein IIb/IIIa blockade compared with heparin and planned glycoprotein IIb/IIIa blockade during percutaneous coronary intervention: REPLACE-2 randomized trial. JAMA 2003;289(7):853–64.

36. O'Gara P, Kuchner F, Ascheim D, et al. 2013 ACCF/AHA guideline for the management of ST-elevation myocardial infarction: a report of the American College of Cardiology Foundation/American Heart Association Task Force on Practice Guidelines. Circulation 2013;127:e362–425.

37. Yusuf S, Zhao F, Mehta SR, et al. Effects of clopidogrel in addition to aspirin in patients with acute coronary syndromes without ST-segment elevation. N Engl J Med 2001;345(7):494–502.

38. Mehta SR, Yusuf S, Peters RJ, et al. Effects of pretreatment with clopidogrel and aspirin followed by long-term therapy in patients undergoing percutaneous coronary intervention: the PCI-CURE study. Lancet 2001;358:527–33.

39. Sabatine M, Cannon C, Gibson M, et al. Addition of clopidogrel to aspirin and fibrinolytic therapy for myocardial infarction with ST-segment elevation. N Engl J Med 2005;352:1179–89.

40. Steinhubl S, Berger PB, Mann J, et al. Early and sustained dual oral antiplatelet therapy following percutaneous coronary intervention a randomized controlled trial. JAMA 2002;288:2411–20.

41. Montalescot G, Bolognese L, Dudek D, et al. Pretreatment with prasugrel in non–ST-segment elevation acute coronary syndromes. N Engl J Med 2013;369:999–1010.

42. Wiviott S, Braunwald E, Mc Cabe C, et al. Prasugrel versus clopidogrel in patients with acute coronary syndromes. N Engl J Med 2009;357:2001–15.

43. Dalby A, Wiviott S, Muprhy S, et al. The influence of the arterial access site and its management on bleeding events in acute coronary syndromes in TRITON - TIMI 38. Circulation 2008;118:638.

44. Wallentin L, Becker R, Budaj A, et al. Ticagrelor versus clopidogrel in patients with acute coronary syndromes. N Engl J Med 2009;361:1045–57.

45. Windecker S, Kolh P, Alfonso F, et al. 2014 ESC/EACTS guidelines on myocardial revascularization. Eur Heart J 2014;35:2541–619.

46. De Luca L, Leonardi S, Cavallini C, et al. Contemporary antithrombotic strategies in patients with acute coronary syndrome admitted to cardiac care units in Italy: the EYESHOT study. Eur Heart J Acute Cardiovasc Care 2014. [Epub ahead of print].

47. Muñiz-Lozano A, Rollini F, Franchi F, et al. Update on platelet glycoprotein IIb/IIIa inhibitors: recommendations for clinical practice. Ther Adv Cardiovasc Dis 2013;7(4):197–313.

48. Kastrati A, Mehili J, Schuhlen H, et al, Intracoronary Stenting Antithrombotic Regimen-Rapid Early Action for Coronary Treatment Study. A clinical trial of abciximab in elective percutaneous coronary

intervention after pretreatment with clopidogrel. N Engl J Med 2004;67(1):21–5.

49. Bosch X, Marrugat J, Sanchis J. Platelet glycoprotein IIb/IIIa blockers during percutaneous coronary intervention and as the initial medical treatment of non-ST segment elevation acute coronary syndromes. Cochrane Database Syst Rev 2013;(11):CD002130.

50. Sciahbasi A, Pristipino C, Ambrosio G, et al. Arterial access-site–related outcomes of patients undergoing invasive coronary procedures for acute coronary syndromes (from the ComPaRison of Early Invasive and Conservative Treatment in Patients With Non–ST-ElevatiOn Acute Coronary Syndromes [PRESTO-ACS] Vascular Substudy). Am J Cardiol 2009;103:796–800.

51. Eichhofer J, Horlick E, Ivanov J, et al. Decreased complication rates using the transradial compared to the transfemoral approach in percutaneous coronary intervention in the era of routine stenting and glycoprotein platelet IIb/IIIa inhibitor use: a large single-center experience. Am Heart J 2008;156(5): 864–70.

52. Collet JP, Huber K, Cohen M, et al. A direct comparison of intravenous enoxaparin with unfractionated heparin in primary percutaneous coronary intervention (from the ATOLL Trial). Am J Cardiol 2013;112:1367–72.

53. Bernat I, Horak D, Stasek J, Mates M, Pesek J, Ostadal P, et al. ST-elevation myocardial infarction treated by RADIAL or femoral approach in a multicenter randomized clinical trial: the STEMI-RADIAL trial. J Am Coll Cardiol 2014;63:964–72.

54. Kiemeneij F, Laarman GJ, Odekerken D, et al. A randomized comparison of percutaneous transluminal coronary angioplasty by the radial, brachial and femoral approaches: the access study. J Am Coll Cardiol 1997;29(6):1269–75.

55. Sanmartin M, Cuevas D, Goicolea J, et al. Vascular complications associated with radial artery access for cardiac catheterization. Rev Esp Cardiol 2004; 57(6):581–4.

56. Bertrand OF, Larose E, Rodes-Cabau J, et al. Incidence, predictors, and clinical impact of bleeding after transradial coronary stenting and maximal antiplatelet therapy. Am Heart J 2009;157(1):164–9.

57. Kanei Y, Kwan T, Nakra NC, et al. Transradial cardiac catheterization: a review of access site complications. Catheter Cardiovasc Interv 2011;78(6):840–6.

58. Spaulding C, Lefevre T, Funck F, et al. Left radial approach for coronary angiography: results of a prospective study. Cathet Cardiovasc Diagn 1996; 39(4):365–70.

59. Plante S, Cantor WJ, Goldman L, et al. Comparison of bivalirudin versus heparin on radial artery occlusion after transradial catheterization. Catheter Cardiovasc Interv 2010;76(5):654–8.

60. Stella PR, Kiemeneij F, Laarman GJ, et al. Incidence and outcome of radial artery occlusion following transradial artery coronary angioplasty. Cathet Cardiovasc Diagn 1997;40(2):156–8.

61. Honda T, Fujimoto K, Miyao Y, et al. Access site-related complications after transradial catheterization can be reduced with smaller sheath size and statins. Cardiovasc Interv Ther 2012;27(3):174–80.

62. Cubero JM, Lombardo J, Pedrosa C, et al. Radial compression guided by mean artery pressure versus standard compression with a pneumatic device (RACOMAP). Catheter Cardiovasc Interv 2009; 73(4):467–72.

63. Sanmartin M, Gomez M, Rumoroso JR, et al. Interruption of blood flow during compression and radial artery occlusion after transradial catheterization. Catheter Cardiovasc Interv 2007;70(2):185–9.

64. Pancholy S, Coppola J, Patel T, et al. Prevention of radial artery occlusion-patent hemostasis evaluation trial (PROPHET study): a randomized comparison of traditional versus patency documented hemostasis after transradial catheterization. Catheter Cardiovasc Interv 2008;72(3):335–40.

65. Politi L, Aprile A, Paganelli C, et al. Randomized clinical trial on short-time compression with Kaolin-filled pad: a new strategy to avoid early bleeding and subacute radial artery occlusion after percutaneous coronary intervention. J Interv Cardiol 2010;24(1):65–72.

66. Pancholy SB, Bertrand OF, Patel T. Comparison of a priori versus provisional heparin therapy on radial artery occlusion after transradial coronary angiography and patent hemostasis (from the PHARAOH Study). Am J Cardiol 2012;110(2):173–6.

67. Bernat I, Bertrand OF, Rokyta R, et al. Efficacy and safety of transient ulnar artery compression to recanalize acute radial artery occlusion after transradial catheterization. Am J Cardiol 2011;107(11): 1698–701.

68. Uhlemann M, Mobius-Winkler S, Mende M, et al. The Leipzig prospective vascular ultrasound registry in radial artery catheterization: impact of sheath size on vascular complications. JACC Cardiovasc Interv 2012;5(1):36–43.

69. Abdelaal E, Molin P, Plourde G, et al. Successive transradial access for coronary procedures: experience of Quebec Heart-Lung Institute. Am Heart J 2013;165(3):325–31.